BYE-BYE CHARLIE

Corinne Manning is an oral historian.
Her previous publications, including the
co-authored book, *A Man of All Tribes:
The Life of Alick Jackomos*, explore issues
of human rights, colonialism, identity and
diversity in Australia. She is currently
working as a research fellow in the School
of Social Sciences at Victoria University.

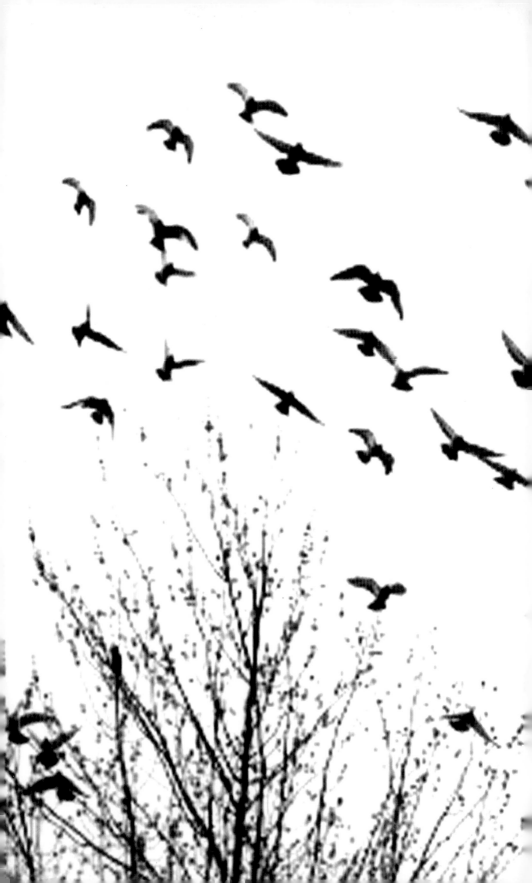

CORINNE MANNING

BYE-BYE CHARLIE
Stories from the Vanishing World of Kew Cottages

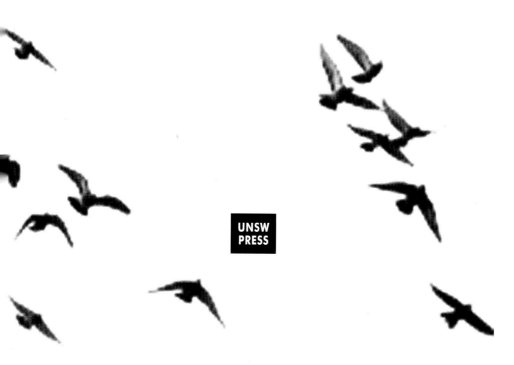

UNSW
PRESS

This history is dedicated to my husband, John,
and to my parents, Alan and Therese.

A UNSW Press book

Published by
University of New South Wales Press Ltd
University of New South Wales
Sydney NSW 2052
AUSTRALIA
www.unswpress.com.au

© Corinne Manning 2008
First published 2008

National Library of Australia
Cataloguing-in-Publication entry
Manning, Corinne.
Bye-bye Charlie: stories from the vanishing world of Kew Cottages/
author, Corinne Manning.
Sydney: University of New South Wales Press, 2008.
ISBN: 978 1 921410 10 9 (pbk.)
Includes index.
Bibliography.

Kew Cottages (Kew, Vic.) – History. Children with mental disabilities –
Institutional care – Victoria – Kew – History. People with mental
disabilities – Institutional care – Victoria – Kew – History. People
with mental disabilities – Services for – Victoria – Kew – History.

362.385099451

Design and cover photo montage Di Quick
Cover includes Edward Rowe, aged four, taken on
admission to Kew Cottages 1925 (courtesy of the
Department of Human Services, Victoria)

Printer Everbest, China.

Contents

Foreword

Many of the institutions of the 20th century, once so dominant, have closed and their land sold for the development of houses. The walls and buildings that for many years defined and contained the lives of tens of thousands of people with intellectual disabilities are being dismantled. What happens then? Who will remember what happened to the people who lived or worked in those places or whose lives – as parents or other family members – were touched by them in profound ways? When the institutions have closed, and the walls have finally come down, there may be little left in the landscape to show what was once there.

This is where oral history becomes vital. It is the means by which the stories of people connected with institutions can be collected and preserved. These stories may become the only lasting and true record of what really happened. We need these stories; without them the events of the 20th century, including the rise and decline of the long-stay institutions, will not be told in all its detail and richness.

Kew Cottages opened in 1887 with high ideals. Its closure follows a harrowing and tragic fire in 1996. But Kew's history, and the histories of the thousands of people who lived and worked there, will not be forgotten. This book guarantees that. In listening to and recording as many stories as possible from those still alive and able to contribute, Corinne Manning has ensured that Kew's history will be preserved forever. In this meticulously researched book, the voices of people with intellectual disabilities are heard and celebrated. This in itself is rare enough. But the book has enabled many other people to bear witness too, and to have their memories included; a rare mix of family voices, ward staff, volunteers, social workers and many other people whose lives were intertwined with the unfolding story of Kew Cottages.

This book tells it all: celebrating what was good and acknowledging the happy memories, but never shirking from or hiding the sadness and unhappiness of many of the people who lived at Kew. This book rescues what otherwise would have remained a hidden history, and sheds light on otherwise 'forgotten lives'.

The site of Kew Cottages is still there, in that leafy suburb of Melbourne. Many of the buildings remain standing, looking the worse for wear (and neglected) and the covered walkway – rusting somewhat – still links them. I know this because I was lucky enough to visit Kew with Corinne Manning (and historian Lee-Ann Monk) during 2007. We took a walk around the grounds and I tried to imagine what it must have been like to live or work there. Already there is little to show for all that happened over the 120 or so years of Kew's existence; so this book does the impossible, it brings Kew Cottages back to life. It also reminds us of the importance of our learning the lessons from history; for in George Santayana's words, 'Those who cannot remember the past are condemned to repeat it.'

Professor Dorothy Atkinson
Open University, United Kingdom

Acknowledgments

In 2005, when I started working on the Kew Cottages History Project, I could never have envisaged the enormous amount of support and encouragement that I have received from so many people throughout my two years of research. The following is a selection of people whom I wish to personally thank, but there are many more that I can not name, due to their wish to remain anonymous.

Firstly, I would like to thank all of the oral history interviewees, the majority of whom are listed in the notes. Your generosity in sharing such personal stories has made for a unique account of institutional living. A great many people also assisted in organising and facilitating interview sessions. In particular, I wish to acknowledge the following people: Tess Blumhoff, Philip Brady, Andrew Cross, members of the Dickson family, particularly Rosemary, Mandy and Daryl, John Foster, Lois Lockwood, Doxia Monev, Elizabeth Mullavey, Judy Osborne, Paul and Margaret Rodgers, and Andrew Slevin. I also wish to recognise the important role that residents' families, friends and direct care staff had in offering photographs and information to be used for the Project. I am grateful to Hilary Johnson, the communication strategist for the History Project, for her advice in making the interview sessions both productive and fulfilling for some interview participants. Amanda Rooke was also vital in transcribing most interviews.

The Kew Cottages History Project was instigated through funding support provided by La Trobe University, Kew Residential Services (KRS)/Victorian Department of Human Services (DHS) and the Australian Research Council through its Linkage Grant scheme. KRS also funded the production of the DVD. I am especially thankful to Alma Adams, Kerrie Soraghan and Maria Heenan for recognising the value of this resource. Simon Westaway, Margaret Purdam and Tim Jessel provided professional skills and advice in relation to producing the collection of digital histories. I would like to acknowledge the generous grants made by Dame Elisabeth Murdoch and Interact Australia which enabled the production of a history that is accessible for people with intellectual disability.

Not only did KRS and DHS offer monetary support, staff members were crucial in providing research assistance and guidance throughout the Project. Once again, I would like to thank Alma Adams, Kerrie Soraghan and Maria Heenan, as well as Istarlin Omar and Ginny Adams.

I owe an enormous debt to fellow members of the Kew Cottages History Project at La Trobe University. One of my greatest pleasures has been working alongside Lee-Ann Monk who offered friendship, intellectual discussion and debate, sage advice and a steady supply of Baci and Haigh's chocolates. Lee-Ann's dedication to the History Project and the welfare of her colleagues has been admirable. I am forever grateful for her support, particularly when dealing with difficult and confronting issues associated with Kew's history. Similarly, I would like to express my appreciation to Chris Dew and John Tebbutt who not only provided support, but also creative inspiration to produce outcomes that were both meaningful and accessible for Kew residents. In addition, Chris Bigby, Richard Broome and Katie Holmes were also instrumental in helping me to conceptualise, facilitate and complete the oral history. The final two members of the research team, Yvonne Ward and Cameron Rose, were also incredibly supportive in supplying materials, feedback and advice on a range of issues.

I am appreciative of the help received from people in the following organisations: Department of Human Services (Records Services) (Vic), Kew Cottages Historical Society, Kew Cottages Parents' Association, National Archives of Australia, National Library of Australia, Public Record Office of Victoria, Royal Melbourne Hospital Library, State Library of Victoria and Victoria Police. I also wish to thank individuals who donated personal papers and documents. I would like to recognise the archival contributions made by Fran van Brummelen, Beryl Power, John Cosmas, Andrea Eve, Louise Godwin, Astrid Judge and Selga Judge. Also, the networking and research support given by David Ballek, Terry Claven and John Kelleher of the Victoria Police, and Ronald Haines of the Metropolitan Fire Brigade (Melbourne).

The images used in *Bye-Bye Charlie* were donated or bought from a variety of sources. Many thanks to Lucas Carter and Rachel McLeod of Fairfax Media Ltd, who not only organised copyright and reproduction, but supplied photocopies of newspaper articles that accompanied images. Tess Flynn and Erin Hartwig, from Photography and Digital Imaging at La Trobe University, were instrumental in reproducing hundreds of images. Thanks are also extended to the Victoria Police for allowing me to use crime scene photos and videos of the 1996 fire for research and publication purposes.

Many people read part or all of the manuscript and offered constructive criticism to enhance the publication. These people included members of the La Trobe research team and KRS, as well as individuals Professor Dorothy Atkinson from the Open University (UK), Bill Westgarth, and members of my family – John Manning, Alan and Therese West and Noreen O'Brien.

Thanks are also due to the team at UNSW Press, particularly Elspeth Menzies and Phillipa McGuinness, who realised the importance of this history and embraced the innovative nature of the publication. Your advice and encouragement were welcomed.

Also to my editor, Jessica Perini, who made the editing process a painless and rewarding experience.

To my friends and colleagues at La Trobe University, I am grateful for the camaraderie that you have offered. Staff room lunches, corridor conversations and laughter were welcomed respite. I am also indebted to Susan Aykut, Janet Butler, Emma Christopher, Lisa McKinney and Sue Taffe for taking an interest in my work, listening to my problems and offering encouragement. You are all true friends.

Lastly, I would like to acknowledge my family. You have all shared my journey into Kew's tumultuous history. In particular, I am indebted to my husband, John, parents, Alan and Therese, and aunty, Noreen, who not only listened to my experiences and stories, but also read the manuscript as it emerged. Your observations, advice and proofreading helped to shape the final history. I am also eternally grateful to my siblings and their families: Nicolas, Simone, Monique, Marcelle, Jerome, Kieran, Helen, Simon, Colin, Briana, James, Sienna, Joshua, Callum, Aidan and Ella. Having worked on this history, I have come to further appreciate the value of family, as many residents that I spoke with craved such interaction with their relatives. You are all inspirational people whom I greatly admire and respect.

Timeline

1887 Kew Idiot Asylum opened (commonly known as Kew Cottages)

1924 Royal Commission held into the conditions at Kew Cottages

1925 Edward (Ted) Rowe admitted, transferred from the Children's Welfare Department, Receiving Depot, Royal Park

1929 First Education Department Special School opened onsite

1933 *Mental Hygiene Act* passed by Victorian Parliament

1934 *Mental Hygiene Act* proclaimed

1937 Coronial Inquest concludes that overcrowding is a key contributor to the death of resident, Thelma Ada Hills

1937 Over 200 residents transferred to alternate State training facilities such as Janefield in Bundoora

1941 Lois Philmore admitted, transferred from a local orphanage, sent to Janefield in 1942

1950 *Mental Hygiene Authority Act* passed by Victorian Parliament

1952 *Mental Hygiene Authority Act* enacted

1952 Appointment of Dr Eric Cunningham Dax as chairman of the newly established Mental Hygiene Authority. Cunningham Dax introduces reforms to improve mental health services in Victoria

1952 Appointment of Irena Higgins as Kew Cottages first social worker. Irena creates an official waiting list for the Cottages and promotes greater family involvement with the institution, particularly by facilitating the establishment of the Kew Cottages Parents' Association

1953 Tipping Appeal, spearheaded by journalist Bill Tipping of the *Herald* newspaper, raises money to renovate dilapidated buildings at Kew. Money raised through the public appeal is matched pound for pound by the Victorian Government

1955 First Occupational Therapy Centre opened through money raised by the Lions Club and Pamplin-Green bequest. Additional training offered to residents through the kindergarten, therapy sessions and industrial workshop

1956 Patrick Reed admitted, transferred from St Augustine's Orphanage (Geelong)

1957 Kew Cottages Parents' Association formed

1957 Kew Cottages administratively separated from Kew Mental Hospital

1958 David Honner admitted, transferred from Pleasant Creek, Stawell

1959 Raymond Bouker admitted

1959 *Mental Health Act* passed by Victorian Parliament enabling residents to be admitted to the Cottages on a voluntary basis, rather than being committed as 'insane', not operative until 1962

1959 Paediatric Unit opened

1961 First Kew Cottages Annual Fete

1962 Wendy Pennycuick and Steven Wears admitted. Wendy is transferred from the Royal Victorian Institute for the Blind

1964 Patricia Rodgers admitted and Lois Philmore re-admitted, transferred from Janefield

1965 Ralph Dawson, John Goddard and Andrew Ledwidge admitted. John is transferred from Spastic Society of Victoria facility

1967 Commonwealth Government introduces the Sheltered Employment Allowance

1967 Kew Cottages Parents' Association takes over responsibility for running the onsite kiosk. Officially named the 'Brady Kiosk'

1968 Donald Starick admitted, transferred from Pleasant Creek, Stawell

1969 Nick Konstantaras admitted

1975 Minus Children Appeal spearheaded by Val Smorgon, Lillian Frank and *The Age* newspaper. The appeal raises $1 million that is matched by an equal sum from the Victorian Government. This results in the construction of activity centres for residents

1977 Opening of the 'Minus Children's buildings' (called Age/Geiger, Hamer, Perkin and Smorgon)

1977 Report of the Victorian Committee on Mental Retardation recommends a shift away from institutional care for people with intellectual disability and for service to be based upon the principles of normalisation

1982 Report of the Minister's Committee on Rights and Protective Legislation for Intellectually Handicapped Persons (Cocks Report) contributed to the formulation of the *Guardianship and Administration Board Act* 1986

1984 First stage of deinstitutionalisation as St Nicholas is closed and residents relocate into community housing

1984 Report of the Committee on the Legislative Framework for

Services to People with Intellectual Disabilities (Rimmer Report). Recommendations are made to devise new legislation to replace the 1959 *Mental Health Act*

1986 *Intellectually Disabled Persons' Services Act* passed by Victorian Parliament, primarily based upon the Rimmer Report

1992 James Barry Woods admitted, transferred from Caloola, Sunbury

1995 Kew Cottages Parents' Association sue the Victorian Government for failing in its duty of care to meet the regulations stipulated by the 1986 Act

1996 Fire in Unit 31 kills nine male residents

1996 Hirondelle Improved Lifestyle Project is instituted, 40 residents who lost their accommodation in the fire are moved into seven community-based group homes between April 1996 and April 1998

1997 Coroner's findings handed down into the fire and deaths of nine men at Kew Cottages on 8 April 1996

1999 Community Relocation Project – 58 residents are relocated into community housing

2001 Closure and redevelopment of Kew Cottages announced by Victorian premier, Steve Bracks

2002 First group of residents relocated into an offsite community residential unit as part of Kew's closure

2005 Closure of the Brady Kiosk

2006 Last group of residents earmarked for relocation to offsite community residential units move to a nearby suburb

2006 *Disability Act* passed by Victorian Parliament

2007 100 residents remain living onsite at Kew until their community residential units are available in 2008

Introduction

What it meant to people like myself, what it meant to people like [my son] Paul, and what it means to so many Victorians that have had something to do with Kew Cottages ... that history should be preserved.

Bill Westgarth, Kew parent, 19 January 2006

The subject of this book emerged from fears expressed by many people, such as Bill Westgarth, that the closure of Kew Cottages would result in the loss of its history. But how was that history to be portrayed? From 2005 to 2007, I was the oral historian on a project undertaken by a team of researchers at La Trobe University to document the history of Kew Cottages. My role was to write a history based upon the memories of people intimately associated with Kew; residents, family, staff, volunteers, administrators, policy makers, emergency service personnel, advocates and visitors. Many staff and families connected with Kew urged me to write about the positive aspects of its history. They wanted the generous support of particular individuals and organisations to be recognised, medical advances and research to be highlighted, and the care shown by particular staff members to be acknowledged. These people did not want a whitewash, but felt aggrieved by all of the 'bad press' that Kew had received over the years. Positive accounts have been noted throughout the history. However, testimony, particularly interviews recorded with residents, have revealed that life at Kew was often challenging. The following recollections provide a rare understanding of the experience of institutional living.

Kew Cottages was Australia's first purpose-built institution for people who were diagnosed with what is now referred to as 'intellectual disability'. When it opened in 1887, Kew was regarded as a world-leading facility as it offered both residential care and educational opportunities. Located in a leafy Melbourne suburb and isolated on a hillside, the site was approximately eight kilometres from the city centre. The institution was constructed adjacent to Kew Lunatic Asylum, later known as Kew Mental Hospital, then Willsmere. At first, these facilities were connected, not only by their close proximity to one another, but also administratively. Initially, they fell under the jurisdiction of the Victorian Government department, Hospitals for the Insane, which established and maintained institutions for the care and treatment of people with intellectual disability and people experiencing 'mental illness'. Throughout its history, Kew Cottages has been known by many names, including Kew Idiot Asylum, Children's Cottages Kew and Kew Residential Services. People closely connected with the institution most commonly refer to it as 'Kew Cottages', 'the Cottages' and simply 'Kew'. Consequently, these three names are used interchangeably in this history.

Kew was developed and managed according to popular notions in the 19th and 20th centuries, that medical professionals were best placed to run these types of institutions. According to academics, Colin Barnes and Geoff Mercer, this practice stemmed from a belief that medicine could 'curb', 'train' or 'cure' the perceived 'problem' of intellectual disability.[1] For nearly a century, medical staff were primarily responsible for overseeing the daily operation of Kew. However, in the 1970s, new philosophies associated with intellectual disability emerged that radically transformed Kew's management. A more multidisciplinary approach to care was implemented combining the skills of medical, health and education specialists. Despite this shift in philosophies, the nature of life at Kew remained regimented, collective and often impersonal.

Kew Cottages was separated from Kew Lunatic Asylum by a picket fence. Originally, in 1887, centralised buildings included the school, kitchen and baths. On one side of these buildings were two single-storey cottages, erected for male residents, on the opposite side was a cottage built for female residents. Over the following decades, many more buildings were constructed to house increasing numbers of residents. These were located separate from, but within the vicinity of the initial cottages. A sheltered walkway was erected which linked various buildings thereby creating a sense of connectedness and unity. In 1887, 40 males and 17 females were accommodated in the new facility.[2] By 1968, the population figure peaked at 948. Kew Cottages had grown to be Australia's largest institution for people with intellectual disability.

Kew Cottages circa 1900, Kew Lunatic
Asylum pictured in the background,
photographer Nicholas Caire.
(Courtesy of Kew Residential Services,
Department of Human Services,
Victoria)

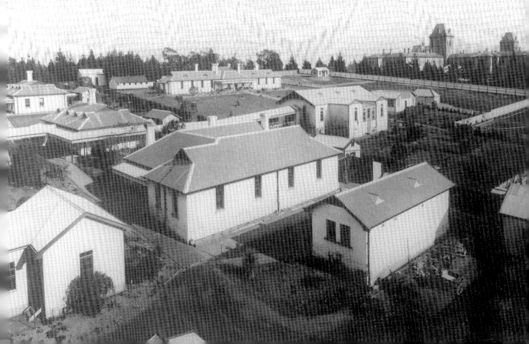

Kew Cottages population statistics by decade from 1887–2007

Year	Total
1887	57
1897	214
1907	292
1917	326
1927	410
1937	500
1947	459
1957	720
1967	946
1977	894
1987	748
1997	547
2007	101

Prior to the early 1960s, residents were committed under Victorian legislation that applied to both people with 'mental illness' and intellectual disability. This system required two doctors to certify an individual as being of 'unsound mind'. Certified people were considered to be 'insane' and in need of custodial State care. In 1959, the Victorian Government passed the *Mental Health Act*. In 1962, the new legislation became operative and allowed for residents to be voluntarily admitted to the Cottages. According to Kew's superintendent, Dr Wilfrid Brady, legislative change was welcomed by many parents and doctors who found it abhorrent to declare a baby or young child 'insane'.[3]

For much of Kew's history, medical professionals categorised and grouped residents according to their varying intellectual and sometimes physical disabilities. Residents were housed in living spaces assigned numerical identification, such as 'Ward 33', but at various times alternate names were used including 'Nursery', 'Schoolboys' and 'Dependent' wards. Within some wards further delineations were made based upon skills' level. For example, terms such as 'big boys', 'small boys', 'high' or 'low' functioning were commonplace. Classification systems not only reflected popular medical practice, but contributed to the appearance of Kew being an ordered institution that catered for the specific needs of residents.

The language and classifications used throughout this history reflect contemporary ideas and attitudes towards people with intellectual disability. In the 21st century some earlier terminology is considered to be highly offensive, however it serves as a valuable tool for understanding the ways in which people formerly spoke about and understood intellectual disability. I have chosen to use 'people-first language' which reflects current international trends and which positions the person as the primary subject, not the perceived disability.[4] Aside from direct quotes, the term 'resident', rather than 'patient' or 'client', has been used to refer to people who were committed and admitted to the Cottages.

Recording oral histories for this project has been extraordinary. My previous experience in the field of Indigenous history proved to be invaluable in preparing for the emotional rollercoaster that is Kew's history. Many interviewees openly wept or showed outward signs of distress when recounting particular stories of hardship, grief or turmoil. At other times there was uproarious laughter and even the odd singalong as happy reminiscences were shared. Working on the Kew Cottages History Project has reinforced the basic tenets of good oral history practice; that in all interview situations establishing an environment of trust, understanding and mutual respect will generally result in positive outcomes for participants.

I was fortunate in being able to locate interviewees who represented a range of eras and roles associated with Kew. The boy pictured on the front cover was the oldest resident interviewed, Ted

Rowe. The photograph was taken on his admission to Kew Cottages in 1925, when he was four years old. While Ted's memories provide a colourful account of life at Kew in the 1920s and '30s, most of the oral history dates from the 1950s to 2007. A variety of recruitment methods were used to secure interviewees including publicity campaigns, mail-outs, word-of-mouth and recommendations from organisations and individuals. Successful recruitment strategies resulted in over 80 people being involved in recording approximately 100 hours of oral history. A focus group with six community visitors from the Office of the Public Advocate, a statutory body responsible for overseeing the welfare of people with disabilities, was also recorded. As particular members of the group wished to remain anonymous all of the testimony from this session has been referred to as coming from 'community visitors'.

In order to provide a history where all interviewees are respectfully acknowledged and their testimony treated as equal, where possible, I have fully named most interviewees, including their title, on the initial reference and used their first, or commonly known name, thereafter. Working against current convention, the surnames of residents have also been used with their consent. This approach gives residents a sense of place and ownership in their history. However, pseudonyms have been chosen by some interviewees because they wish to remain anonymous. Other people were given pseudonyms in order to protect their identity in relation to sensitive information contained in the history. The following is the list of pseudonyms: Anna, James and Michelle Davison, Barry Evans, Liam Ford, Rose Martin and Sean Miller, Caroline Porter, Dianne Pymble, Emily and Melanie Shield, Peter Small, Clare Turner and Michael (Tipping Appeal).

Part I of this history, 'The Journey to Kew', describes the road taken to the Cottages by a range of people whose stories uncover complex and often emotional issues associated with State institutionalisation. For many families and staff, their journey to Kew was a life-defining moment and a significant part of their history with the Cottages. Once at Kew, people were faced with new challenges and experiences. Part II, 'A New World', outlines the multifaceted world that existed within the Cottages. It examines the institution's history from the perspective of residents' experiences and documents the relationships between different people and environments. Part III, 'Leaving Kew', relates some of the ways that residents left the Cottages. It explores a momentous event in Kew Cottages' history, a fire that killed nine men in 1996. It also considers the impact of Kew's closure and redevelopment on people most closely connected with the institution. The inclusion of a collection of digital histories with this book not only brings to life residents' stories, but enables people with limited literacy skills to access the history. Through both the written text and digital histories we glean a unique understanding of life inside one of Australia's most significant institutions.

This history gives voice to some of Australia's most silenced and forgotten people; the residents of Kew Cottages. Although Kew Cottages was founded upon high-minded ideals, persistent overcrowding, inadequate funding and government and public apathy resulted in life being difficult for most residents. *Bye-Bye Charlie* is a testament to the determination and strength of many residents who overcame such adversity. Working with residents has been one of the most rewarding aspects of this history. I have found them to be engaging, insightful and entertaining people. Many of them displayed an acute awareness of the institutional system and offered accounts of how they contravened particular regulations. Residents' testimony also highlighted their willingness and ability to exercise certain powers within Kew to enhance their lives. *Bye-Bye Charlie* is a story of residents' survival within a world of continual deprivation. Their resilience is evident in the self-reflection of one resident in 2006, Ralph Dawson when he stated, 'I'm clever, I use my head … I think positive … I'm happy.'[5]

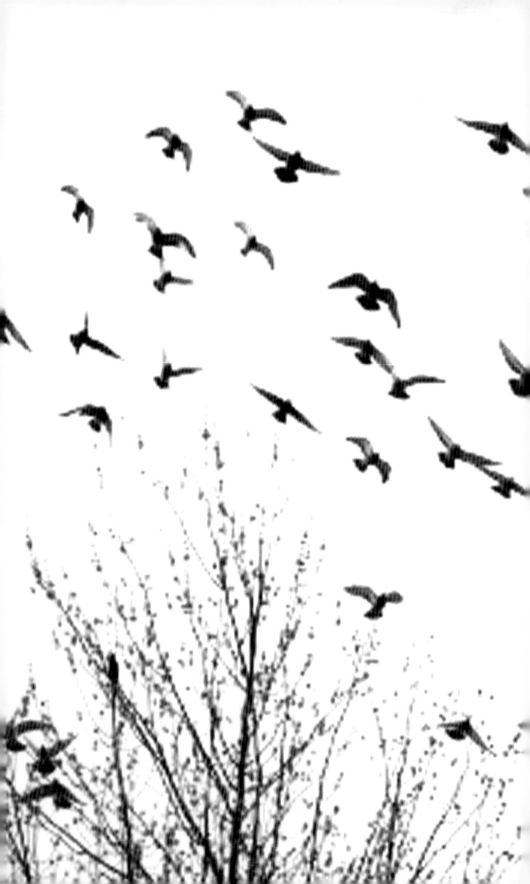

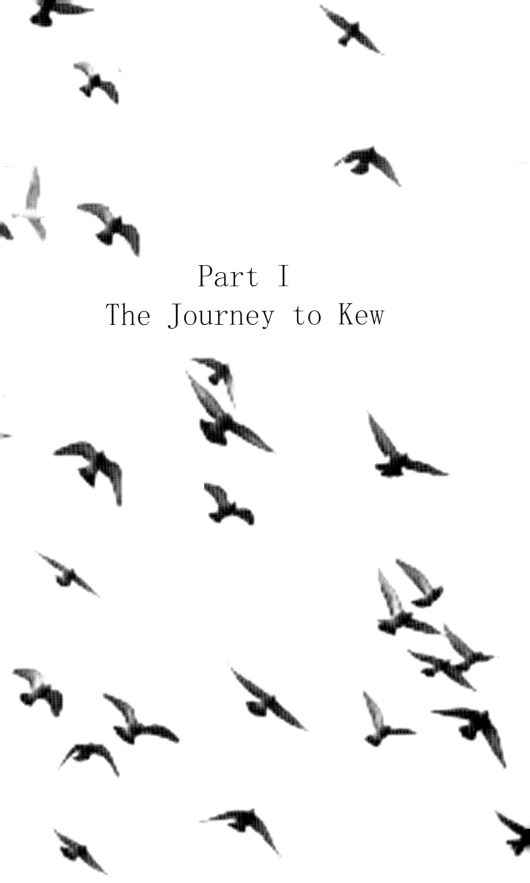

Part I
The Journey to Kew

I had a car accident
I was just hit and knocked by a car
I was sick
I went to hospital to get stitches

1966
40 years ago
I went to Royal Park
I went to Mont Park

[I went to] Sunbury
24 years [in] Sunbury
that's true!

I came to Kew after Sunbury
I had to go to Kew, it [Sunbury] was closing,
remember?
I liked Kew.
James Barry Woods, resident, 8 September
2006 and 15 September 2006

This is how James Barry Woods explains his journey to Kew Cottages. His account was unique in the interviews conducted for this history. James was born in 1934 and grew up in Melbourne with his parents, sister and two brothers. The reason for James' intellectual disability is listed as 'unknown', but a difficult forceps birth was noted by a doctor as a possible cause in his files. At the age of 32, James was admitted to State facilities that housed people with 'mental illness' and people with intellectual disability, Royal Park, Mont Park and Sunbury Mental Training Centre. His admission was prompted by family concerns about James's safety after he ran into an oncoming car travelling on the road outside of his home. When Sunbury was earmarked for closure its residents were relocated. With limited community housing available, some displaced residents were sent to live in other institutions. James was transferred to Kew Cottages in 1992 where he lived for 13 years.

'Can you remember when you first went to Kew?' This question was asked of all interviewees. The resounding answer from

Kew residents was, 'No'. The main reason for this response was that most of the participants were young children aged between three to nine years when they were placed into State care. Patrick Reed and Barry Evans were sent to the Cottages as adults. They were able to list the names of other congregate care facilities where they resided before Kew which included orphanages and hospitals such as St Joseph's (Broadmeadows), St Augustine's (Geelong), Sunbury and Mont Park.[1] Place names were emblazoned on their minds; the experience of getting there was not forthcoming.

Most residents who were interviewed were able to recall precious memories of family life prior to living in institutions. James fondly spoke about his mother cooking pancakes which they ate spread with raspberry jam.[2] Andrew Ledwidge recalled watching his father cutting the grass with his Victa lawnmower in order to keep the snakes away.[3] When telling these stories residents' faces lit up, smiles beamed from ear-to-ear. These brief glimpses reflected the importance that many interviewees placed upon their family history and childhood memories. It was clearly evident that these residents valued the time that they spent living with their families. They were also confident in talking about life in an institution. For residents, it was not the journey to Kew that produced lasting memories, but the experience of living in different worlds.

However for other people intimately associated with Kew, the journey to the Cottages was often a life defining experience. In order to understand the nature of life at Kew Cottages it is essential to understand how people came to visit or work in such a secluded world. The following two chapters describe the various journeys undertaken by people most closely associated with Kew Cottages: families, employees and voluntary workers.

CHAPTER 1

A River of Tears

… through those people of the Children's Cottage [sic] and the doctor I at least came to understand that it is no fault of ours that she came as she did; and to me that meant a lot, as our local doctor had been a little harsh about it. The child died after six weeks at Kew. We don't talk about it among our friends now, as they don't seem to know anything of such sadness in life. So we just go on laughing on the outside and crying on the inside.

'A Country Mother', *Herald*, 5 October 1948

Reluctantly sought, sometimes welcomed, often unexpected, the road to Kew Cottages was a heartbreaking journey for most parents. Although situated in lush parkland, the Cottages lay in the menacing shadow of the 'main building': Kew Mental Hospital. Despite the fact that Kew Cottages was physically separated from the Hospital and granted independent status in 1957, generally people considered them one facility. It was difficult enough for family members to commit their adult relatives to such a forbidding institution, but for many to hand over a child proved almost unbearable. Since 1887 thousands of men and women have sent their children to live at Kew

Cottages. Parents chose this option for various reasons. Many were forced to relinquish their children into State care by circumstances beyond their control, being unable or unwilling to care for children with disabilities at home. Others believed the Cottages offered their children a brighter future with specialised medical services and developmental programs. The following stories primarily focus upon the experiences of parents in the 1940s–60s. These accounts illustrate the complex and often agonising path taken by parents who surrendered their children into State care.

Pregnancy evokes varied responses from expectant parents. Some people are dismayed by the news; they do not wish to bring a child into the world and institutional care facilities were a welcomed option whether their child was disabled or not. For other parents, having to consider institutional care for their newborn was confronting. These parents-to-be had often counted down the months, anxiously awaiting the arrival of their baby, collecting furniture and clothing, preparing a new life for their family. This was certainly the case for one Victorian couple who were elated on the discovery that they were expecting a baby, 'When the baby was coming, how thrilled and excited we were! We planned names and I made all the personal things and clothes, for we felt that nothing we could buy would be good enough.'[1] Jubilation at becoming parents quickly turned to dismay when they were informed of their daughter's intellectual disability:

> Our baby arrived in January, 1947. The doctor who had been our medico since childhood would not allow my husband to tell me for six weeks that the baby we had longed for was a Mongol. I put in six weeks of planning what our daughter would be when she grew up, and imagined what she would wear for years ahead; but in the fifth week after her birth I realised that something was wrong.[2]

Living in country Victoria, the local doctor suggested that the couple consult a specialist in Melbourne:

> Under instructions from our doctor, I took the baby to a Collins Street specialist and there, in his quiet consulting room, he had to

tell me that the child was a Mongol and had a congenital heart which meant that she would not live long. There in Melbourne, from a strange man, I received the most dreadful shock of my life.[3]

Parents in this situation were faced with the unenviable task of deciding on the future care of their children: would or could they look after them at home or should they place them in an institution? In this case the doctor recommended that the baby be sent to Kew. Heart-broken, the parents agreed. Six weeks after committal to the Cottages their daughter passed away.

In Australia today many expectant parents choose to undergo pregnancy tests, such as ultrasound scans, to determine if their unborn children have any detectable congenital problems or abnormalities. These tests were unavailable or rarely used before the late 1960s.[4] Although most expectant parents were undoubtedly worried about the wellbeing of their children, many did not anticipate major problems. The shock of discovering that their children were disabled was often immobilising. On many occasions, parents sought the advice of medical experts to assist them in making the 'right' decision about their children's care.

The role of medical practitioners was often crucial in the parents' decision to place their children at Kew. It was common for parents to be told by doctors to 'forget' about their newborn, to go home and have another baby, or devote themselves to their other child or children.[5] In today's society, such advice appears insensitive, even abhorrent. However, the social conditions in Australia up until the 1970s, particularly the lack of disability support services, made life extremely difficult for parents who chose to look after their children at home. Many medical experts believed that institutional care was in the best interests of the children and their families.

While often the bearer of tragic news, a paediatrician from the Royal Children's Hospital, Dr Elizabeth Turner, was praised by many parents for her compassion and concern for the welfare of families. Rose Miller, whose son was admitted to the Cottages at the age of nine, recalled:

She was very good … [Sean] must have been around about five … when I first ran into her, she said: 'Oh you're going to need a holiday, I'll put his name down on the waiting list at the Kew Cottages' … One day she pulled down my eyelid and she said: 'You're anaemic; you'd better go and get something. It's getting to you.' She wasn't just interested in the patients, she was interested in everything.[6]

The often unquestioning acceptance of medical opinion was not a failing of parents to be proactive in their children's care, but reflected a popular attitude among Australians at that time, that medical specialists 'knew best'.[7]

The recommendation by many medical experts to place children into institutional care resulted from their understanding of the pressures involved in looking after children with disabilities. These pressures sometimes resulted in marital and family breakdown. Fran van Brummelen, a social worker at the Cottages from 1969–94, emphasised this viewpoint. She visited some of the families who were considering placement of their children at Kew. Although a few support services existed in the community, such as day centres and organisations such as the Helping Hand Association, these offered temporary respite. Fran had witnessed the strain that a child with disabilities living at home without adequate services could place on marriages and family life:

It was very frustrating because often when the children came to the Cottages it was a process of: 'Well, it's the only place.' You were always aware that this child should really remain as part of the family, but there weren't the community services to support the child or the family.[8]

In 1957, Irena Higgins, Kew Cottages' first social worker, instigated the formation of the Kew Cottages Parents' Association. The Association encouraged parents to maintain an interest in their children's welfare, even after their placement into institutional care. It also assisted parents who were considering admitting their child to an institution, or were on a waiting list for an institutional place. Association members used a variety of means – regular meetings, information sessions, visits to peoples' homes and publications – to keep parents informed and connected with others in their situation.[9] Rose Miller was grateful for this help:

> Immediately after [Sean] was put onto the waiting list of the Kew Cottages, I got their newsletters. There was a fellow called Mac Brazier who was the editor of the newsletter. He made you feel you're not the only one in this position ... They had a group of people, volunteers, and a lady who came out once a fortnight and watched him for a couple of hours. She sent me off [shopping] to Chadstone! I was getting these newsletters which sort of cheered me up in my hours of horror.[10]

Bill and Joan Westgarth also had dealings with the Association before their son, Paul, went to Kew. In 1966, the Westgarths were approached by Les Jacobs, the Association's president, at an information session they attended about intellectual disability:

> This fellow came over to us, a bloke called Jacobs ... introduced himself, sat down on the ground with us, had a yarn to us about the Parents' Association, about Kew Cottages, and the general problems of being a parent of a handicapped person. He told me that we could join the Parents' Association, it might help ... so we did ... Paul was admitted about seven or eight months later ... [being] able to talk to other people who have similar problems to you, now that's not going to stop the problems, it's not going to make them go away, but at least you can discuss it. I feel that that did Joan a lot of good because she could talk to people who were having the same sort of problems as she was having.[11]

Services offered by the Parents' Association alleviated Bill, Joan and Rose's sense of isolation and despair as they struggled to care for their children at home. For most parents, their journey to Kew Cottages was a lonely experience.

Although some parents were undoubtedly relieved that institutional care was available, as this enabled them to relinquish responsibility for looking after an 'unwanted' child, many others found their hopes and dreams of life with their babies unfulfilled. Parents who chose to immediately place their newborn babies into State care, some permanently severing relationships with their children, were not heartless or selfish, such decisions were often extremely difficult and painful. They would not witness their babies' first

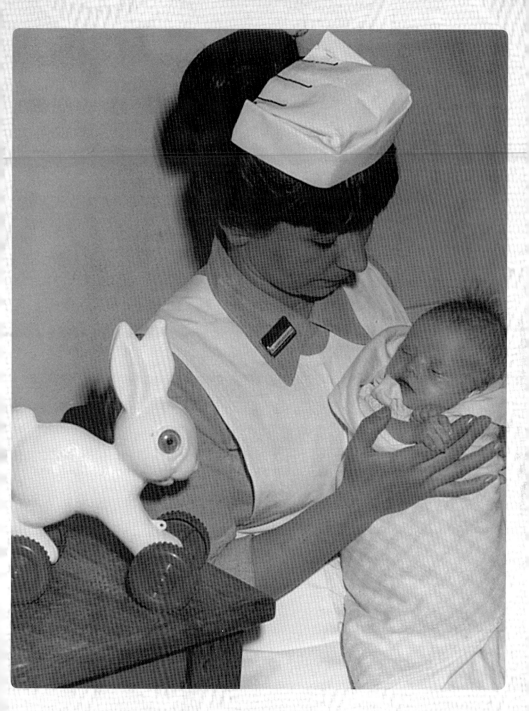

Some residents were admitted to the
Cottages within hours of their birth,
circa 1960. (Courtesy of Cliff Judge,
private collection)

awkward steps, hear their first words or carefully watch them breathe during slumber; their cradles were empty.

In 1962, Joan Jones and her husband were faced with the difficult decision of whether to place their newborn son, Richard, into institutional care after he was diagnosed with Down Syndrome. Joan recalled:

> He was our second child … No two parents could have been less prepared for this event. Neither of us had any personal experience with a seriously disabled person. And so the question of what was the best thing to do for our baby seemed overwhelming. We turned to our doctors who we then believed were experts in these matters. My obstetrician, when asked what was the potential of our child would only say, 'Well, he'll never make a prime minister.' The paediatrician, on the other hand, assured me that this child would never have the emotional development for us to be able to do anything for him and strongly advised placing him in care and concentrating our lives on our seven-year-old daughter … at the time we believed this advice to be sound.[12]

Following the paediatrician's advice, Richard was sent directly from the maternity hospital to a small private infant hospital. Joan was happy with the care that Richard received at his first home, but was critical of the hospital's attitude towards family inclusion. When the matron of the hospital was on duty she refused to allow young siblings into the building. As a result of this restriction, Joan's daughter was forced to wait in the car outside, sometimes peering through a window in order to catch a glimpse of her baby brother.[13] When Richard was six weeks old, a bassinette vacancy became available in the Nursery Ward at Kew and was offered to the Jones family. They accepted this place. Joan remembered the day of his admission:

> I shall always remember that day, when having had two doctors certify our infant son … we committed him to an institution, for as we thought, the rest of his life. We had been to the Cottages earlier to talk to Irena Higgins, the senior social worker at that time, and told ourselves that, with very few alternatives, this was the best thing to do.[14]

Joan stated that Richard's transfer to Kew was a positive experience, 'The family was welcomed as a whole and assured that we were all welcome to visit as often as we wished and to regard our baby's new home as our home too."[15] This inclusive and caring attitude lessened the guilt and sadness Joan felt at committing her child into permanent State care.

Unlike the Jones family, who were aware of Richard's condition from birth, other parents went for weeks, months or years before a diagnosis was made. Symptoms of particular conditions only became apparent over time. This was the case for the Davison family. On 24 November 1953, Anna and James Davison celebrated the birth of their baby girl Michelle. Only months later, these proud parents were devastated by the news that due to physical trauma at birth Michelle was intellectually disabled. Even 53 years later, the Davisons appeared saddened when they described her condition:

ANNA Her brain got squashed and her [motor skills were affected], she thinks all right, but her motivation is wrong and she can't ... [pause]

JAMES ... she can't work her fingers the way she'd like to.[16]

Michelle also began to have epileptic seizures that sometimes resulted in hospitalisation. When James and Anna were told that Michelle's condition was permanent, they elected to continue looking after her at home. As Michelle was one of four children, tending to her daily and medical needs was sometimes overwhelming. Anna commented:

The difficult part was that she was having these terrible fits.
We were up at four o'clock in the morning ... taking her to the
Children's Hospital and waiting in a big long queue for two hours
when Michelle would be running around the place. That was the
worst part, but she was always a loving little girl.[17]

Regular visits to the Children's Hospital were a feature of the Davisons' life as Michelle received treatment for various health problems and was examined by specialist consultants. Many parents who chose to look after their children at home were forced to develop diagnostic and medical expertise to determine when hospital treatment was necessary. This responsibility added to the burden of caring for a child with disabilities.

After witnessing the deterioration of their children's health, and aware of intolerant attitudes held by some members of the community towards people with disabilities, a few parents secretly hoped their children would pass away. Anna Davison expressed this sentiment. At the age of four Michelle had an epileptic seizure and fell into a coma. She was kept alive in hospital via a feeding tube. Weeping gently Anna confided, 'I would have loved her just to pass away as a beautiful little girl, but it wasn't to be!'[18] Some parents experienced this feeling watching their children endure frequent bouts of misery and pain, unable to imagine a fulfilling life or future for their offspring. Michelle recovered from her illness and returned home. Anna, however, remains tormented by her momentary wish for her 'beautiful little girl' to die in peace.

James and Anna first visited Kew Cottages when they decided to place Michelle in respite care in order to spend more quality time with their other children. Anna did not anticipate that this temporary placement would forever change their lives:

> Michelle only went into Kew after they took her in the school holidays, to give me a holiday. [When we went to pick her up] Sister Sue Tomes said: 'No way, how could you look after her? She must come [here], you must part with her and bring her in.'[19]

The power of the Kew medical staff to determine the manner of care for some children with intellectual disability was indicated by the Davisons' simple statement that they, 'did what we were told'.[20] Michelle was admitted to Kew at the age of eight where she lived for over 40 years.

A few months after the birth of their daughter, George and Olive Earl discovered that Lorraine was intellectually disabled. The only indication was a small red mark on the eye, apparently a 'tiny imperfection'. Even the medical experts were unaware of the serious health problems that it forebode. George fondly remembered the birth of his daughter, 'When I saw Lorraine she was ... such a beautiful little compact build. She was very pretty except for this little red mark in the eye.'[21] Nursing staff told George and Olive that the mark was nothing to worry about and sent them home. However, concerned for their daughter, they consulted an eye specialist who had the unenviable task of telling them that the problem was associated with the brain, not the eye.

Lorraine underwent tests at the Children's Hospital which revealed that she had suffered a massive cerebral haemorrhage at birth. Specialists could provide no explanation as to how the haemorrhage occurred, leaving a question that has haunted George for over 50 years. Although no substantive evidence exists to support his claims, George suspects that a medical mishap may have occurred at the hospital, 'In our case we wanted the child, we didn't do a thing wrong and yet Lorraine turned out that way. That's the part that makes me question. I was a policeman, a bit on the suspicious side … I've got no evidence and it's only what I think *might* have happened.'[22] George's need to find a definitive answer for Lorraine's disability was not unusual; this quest to discover whether it was medical negligence or pure bad luck was undertaken by many parents.

George and Olive cared for Lorraine at home until she was six years of age. During these years, their daughter's health gradually deteriorated. George stated that Lorraine looked frail and ill, 'her body withered away. You couldn't imagine how thin she got.'[23] The Earls also struggled with the fact that Lorraine did not reciprocate their affection. She failed to reach the milestones of other children who delighted their parents with their first utterance of 'Mum' or 'Dad'; she did not mirror her mother's smile or giggle when tickled by her father. Lorraine and her parents never enjoyed the formative moments that most parents crave and celebrate during their child's development. George and Olive did not receive even the slightest recognition from Lorraine that she understood their special relationship:

GEORGE Lorraine has never known if we are her parents.

OLIVE Never known. She wouldn't know us as her mother and father.[24]

Life in the Earl household was often trying. Olive bore most of the responsibility for tending to Lorraine's constant needs, as well as looking after her other two children. Being a policeman, George was required to work different shifts and overtime, and his contribution to life at home was sporadic. Olive recollected, 'It became a lot for us to have the other two children and Lorraine who was unable to do anything and would never be able to do anything.'[25] Olive reflected on her other daughter's attitude towards her sister, '[Denise] was only two years older than Lorraine and she'd have her little friends down the street playing ... Lorraine would always be in her pram and she used to call her the "sick little sister".'[26] As Lorraine grew the burden of care increased. The Earls sought advice from their local doctor and were told that their daughter would never improve; she would never walk or talk. On his recommendation, they sent her to live at Kew Cottages. George said that this was not an easy decision, 'It was the worst thing that we reluctantly did, but it was necessary because she's a baby that needed 24-hour treatment.'[27] In 1953, the Earls agreed for Lorraine to be committed to Kew. After the Cottages' closure in 2008, she will continue to live on site in one of the new community residential units.

Physical indicators were not always present in cases of intellectual disability. Many parents only became aware that their child was intellectually disabled when developmental or behavioural issues arose. Hilda Logan and her husband Bob Campbell sought medical advice when their son, Andrew, began to lose some of his speech between two to three years of age. Hilda recalled:

> We went to the obstetrician and she sent us to Dr Elizabeth Turner, the paediatrician, who was very well known. She told us that she felt that Andrew was functioning as though he was mentally retarded ... She then said: 'Don't bankrupt yourselves by going up and down Collins Street looking for another answer. When he needs to be referred to people, I'll refer him.' At that stage Andrew was not looking into our faces at all, he was looking past us, as a lot of people with autism do, and it was as though he was living in his own world. We could let an alarm clock off just near Andrew's ear and he wouldn't even turn around and look to see where the noise came from.[28]

Elizabeth sent Andrew for deafness testing. Once this was ruled out, she recommended that Hilda and Bob enrol Andrew at a kindergarten

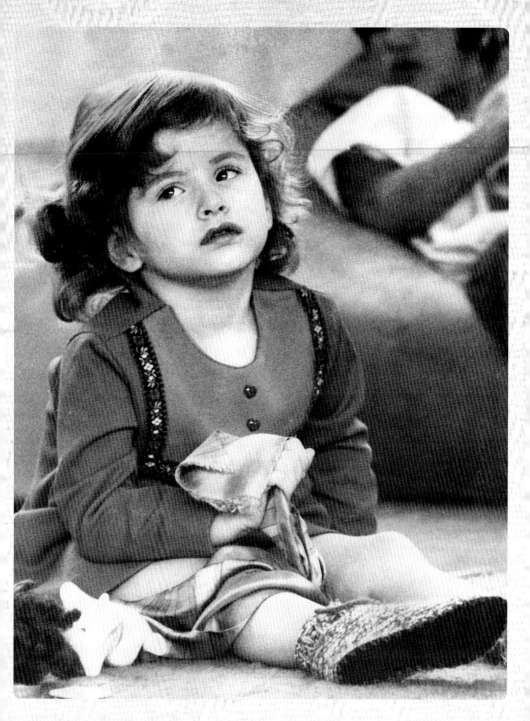

A young resident of Kew Cottages,
1975. (Courtesy of *The Age* Archives/
The Age, Melbourne)

that would meet his special needs. For 12 years, Andrew lived at home and attended the Oakleigh Day Centre. During this time, he was also a short-term resident at Travancore and Kew Cottages as respite for his parents and where he participated in research studies about non-verbal children.

Life for Hilda and Bob was hard. Andrew was an active child who slept little and was prone to escaping. They went to great lengths to protect him:

> Our house was like a fortress. I always had a key to the front door in my pocket as we had to deadlock it to stop him opening it. All of the fences were taken up an extra two feet and we had cyclone gates across the back of the drive. If he got over those, his father had made a magic eye that went over the drive and a hooter sounded in the house as he ran through the beam. When the hooter sounded I would start *running* ... He sure could run![29]

Hilda recalled that on several occasions, she phoned the police to help locate Andrew, 'The police in Moorabbin knew Andrew almost as intimately as we did.'[30]

When Andrew was 11 years old, his father passed away from a congenital heart condition. Hilda had limited family support, one of her sisters helped out as much as she could, but she had three children of her own, and Hilda's mother died nine weeks after Bob. Hilda was fortunate to have neighbours who welcomed her and Andrew into their homes and lives:

> The people that lived in the street were very good to me, particularly one family ... They had a son, David, who was a bit younger than Andrew. David's birthdays were the only ones that Andrew was ever invited to. I was often intrigued with David. All of his little schoolmates would be there, and here was this strange little boy who didn't speak. I used to wait for David to say: 'Oh well, he doesn't talk or anything', but to them he was just Andrew, David didn't feel that he needed to explain him away.

> All of the neighbours were helpful, like using their cars to go out to look for [Andrew]. I had a wonderful family next door and they became almost like [his] grandparents ... They were quite a lot older than me and her elderly mum lived there. She always knitted the

school jumpers for her great grandchildren. At the beginning of the year she would always say to me: 'Hilda, you'd better get the wool for Andrew's school jumpers.' She knitted him two school jumpers every year. They were lovely people. That was the support that I had.[31]

Just over a year after losing her husband Hilda experienced a cancer scare which required major surgery. She was no longer able to care for Andrew alone, so, with a heavy heart, Hilda organised to admit him to Kew, 'I had to have [an] operation. I couldn't leap fences as I had done in the past and run after Andrew. I was just worn out, so that's why he went to Kew.'[32] Andrew was 12 years old. He remained living at Kew until 2005 when he was relocated to community housing at the age of 49.

Rosalie and Eric Trower's experience with their son Stephen was similar to Hilda and Bob's. However they were determined not to commit him to State care. Rosalie recounted:

As a little fellow, of say three, Stephen wasn't talking, and we thought he must be deaf. I knew of the Princess Elizabeth Kindergarten for Deaf Children, in Elgar Road, so I took Stephen up there ... At the end of six months the Directress ... called me in and she said: 'No Rosalie, Stephen isn't deaf, I don't know what his problem is.' Then came the search. I got a lot of literature from America, there was this strange thing called 'autism'.[33] Autism just wasn't a word in Australia.[34]

Rosalie and Eric realised that Stephen's condition was permanent, but resisted sending him to an institution. So, for the first 30 years of his life, Stephen lived at home and in other special accommodation facilities such as Kindilan in Red Hill South. Rosalie explained that an accident at Kindilan set in motion the series of events that resulted in Stephen's admission to Kew:

[Stephen's] job was to carry out the rubbish, and he fell over with the rubbish and knocked his head. They took him inside, he came to and he was all right. They put a bit of mercurochrome on and rang me to say: 'We decided we'd put him into Dromana Hospital, but he's fine.' I think it was just to keep an eye on him. In the afternoon I rang the Dromana Hospital and said who I was, and how was

Stephen? She said: 'Look, he's good, but he's sleeping so we'll leave him here overnight and if you like to come down in the morning you can go back to Kindilan.' I said: 'Oh that's fine.' He wasn't sleeping, he was in a coma. And that was the beginning of terrible times.[35]

Stephen was transferred to the Royal Melbourne Hospital where he underwent major surgery. Rosalie vividly recalled the subsequent sequence of events:

> I remember the surgeon rang me, I was here [at home] on my own of course, and he said: 'I'm going to explain what we'll have to do. We've taken a look inside and we may have to touch part of Stephen's brain, we hope not, but we think we will because oedema has set in. He won't be the same again.' I said: 'Thank you for ringing.' I was just standing there and I thought: 'What do you *do*, who do you pray to, what do you pray for? That he goes out? That he survives?' You don't *know* what to do. Anyway he did survive ... when that was finished there was nowhere for him to go to. He couldn't come home to me, I couldn't give him after-care, Kindilan wasn't equipped for it, so he went out to Larundel. Awful. That's where he nearly died.[36]

Rosalie's friend, Dr Joan Curtis, visited Stephen at Larundel. She reported being appalled by the conditions and said to Rosalie, 'Get him out, he's not going to survive.'[37] It was 1982 and alternate care options were scarce. Desperate for somewhere to accommodate her son, Rosalie went to inspect an institution at Sunbury. Shocked by conditions, which she considered inhumane, Rosalie demanded Stephen be sent to Kew, or she would be forced to take him home. Initially social welfare authorities refused her pleas, but after much lobbying and the threat of drawing media attention to her situation, they acquiesced. Rosalie received a phone call from the chief medical officer at Larundel informing her that Stephen was going to be transferred to Kew Cottages.[38] On the morning of his transfer Rosalie went to Kew with her sister Barby:

> My sister came up from Geelong to be with me ... [we] waited in the car park until we saw Steve going in. I heard him, this high-pitched cry, like a bird, crying: 'Ohawwaa, Ohaaa, Ohaaa' I said: 'Barby, there's Steve, he's going in now.' I felt like a latter-day Judas, that I had *betrayed* my son, I had betrayed *my son*, he'd gone to an institution.[39]

Even though Stephen was a 30-year-old man, the pain and sorrow of placing him in an institution was overwhelming for Rosalie.

A sense of failure was commonplace among many parents who placed their children into institutional care. This was acknowledged by Geoff and Elsie Welchman who began their journey to Kew when their son, David, contracted chicken pox at 11 months and developed encephalitis. Elsie recalled this terrible time:

> He was unconscious in the Children's Hospital for nine days, died twice and was revived, and he's ended up with very bad brain damage. He can't speak, physically he's fit as a fiddle, but mentally he's only about a three or a four year old.[40]

Geoff and Elsie received conflicting advice about the prospect for David's recovery:

ELSIE Dr Powell, and the [people in the] ward that he was in said he would recover, but it'd take five years … Dr Turner [said] there's no way he'll recover, he may not even walk or sit up or anything, unless you can get help for him.

GEOFF At the time Dr Turner said: 'He's a candidate for Kew Cottages, by the time he's eight you'll never manage him, he'll be so hyperactive, disruptive and destructive.' And that's just what he was.

ELSIE When Dr Turner [said] that … I was looking at this little baby and thinking: 'Oh, fancy putting him out into Kew Cottages.' And then Geoff said: 'Well, you don't have to send him now, but we'd better put his name on the waiting list in case we need to, we've got a foot in the door.' So that's what we did. And he went to Kew when he was seven and a half.

GEOFF We hung on for five years hoping that Dr Powell's prognosis would be …

ELSIE The right one.[41]

The Welchman family adjusted to life with a child with disabilities, but it was very challenging. Elsie recalled that leaving the house was often a trial:

> At doctors' surgeries and in the community and on the buses and so on, people would look at you and you could feel they were saying: 'Oh well *she* looks all right, what's wrong with *him*?' That's just how it feels. I remember we'd taken him in to have his eyes tested ... We were left waiting, and of course he didn't wait, David was getting naughty. I gave him the car keys to play with, and [my daughter] Nancy was with me ... he looks at them and just went wild, threw them, and nearly hit a woman. Well, she took to me like nobody's business: 'How *dare* you let a boy behave like that and the little girl's so good' ... I said: 'I'm sorry but he's retarded.' She just went on abusing me, so I got up, took him out, and I said to the girl at the desk: 'I can't sit in there any longer with David, he's just impossible.' I said that people were getting annoyed with me for letting him misbehave. So she put me straight in, which was good, but that's the sort of thing that happened.[42]

The pressure felt by many parents was compounded by the intolerance shown by some people in the general community towards people with intellectual disability.

As the years went by the ramifications of living with a child with disabilities took their toll on family life in the Welchman household. Geoff recognised the hardship felt by his wife and their three other children, 'It was very much to their disadvantage and they couldn't sleep, couldn't study, and he was going to destroy their life and Elsie's health.'[43] There were also security concerns, as David would sometimes run off:

GEOFF We had six foot high cyclone extensions on the fence all round.

ELSIE He just used to hop over them like a kangaroo, and off! He ... used to get miles away in no time at all. Then one night he got over at the corner of Warrigal and Centre Roads ...

GEOFF Running across the traffic.

ELSIE Yes running through the traffic, at five o'clock at night.

GEOFF No road-sense at all. I thought that he should go to Kew for his own safety ... by the time he was seven years of age we decided that for the sake of everybody, and his own sake, Kew Cottages was the place for him.[44]

The rollercoaster journey endured by the Welchmans was experienced by many parents who clung to the hope that their child would develop sufficiently to continue living at home.

David's admission to Kew was a harrowing experience:

ELSIE It was the hardest thing we ever did, we felt he'd been thrown to the lions ... the nurse came to get him to take him down to the units, and said: 'Is that David?' and I said: 'Yes' and she said: 'He can't come to our unit, he's too small, it's a school ward. He'll get his teeth knocked down his throat.' ... We went to see Dr Brady [the superintendent of the Cottages] and he was having Christmas dinner, he wasn't there, so we brought him home ... [Dr Brady rang us and] said: 'Oh, bring him back, straight away, he's on our register now, we're responsible for him.' I said: 'Well he's not going where he was put in the first place.' He said: 'No, I'll put him in another unit altogether.'

GEOFF To park him there and drive away was very, very hard.[45]

Even though the Welchmans made a rational decision in the best interests of all family members, they were emotionally devastated at entrusting David into the care of strangers at Kew. Geoff and Elsie were acutely aware that in committing David their parental rights were extinguished. Legally they were powerless to make decisions about his future care.

In rare cases, childhood inoculation resulted in children suffering from permanent disability. This was the case for Bill and Joan Westgarth who found themselves on the road to Kew with their son, Paul. Bill explained:

We lived in Malaya ... he was born in 1963, and in about January 1964 he started having long seizures, status epilepsy. The first one of these, the status part of it, lasted for about 30 hours, and he finished

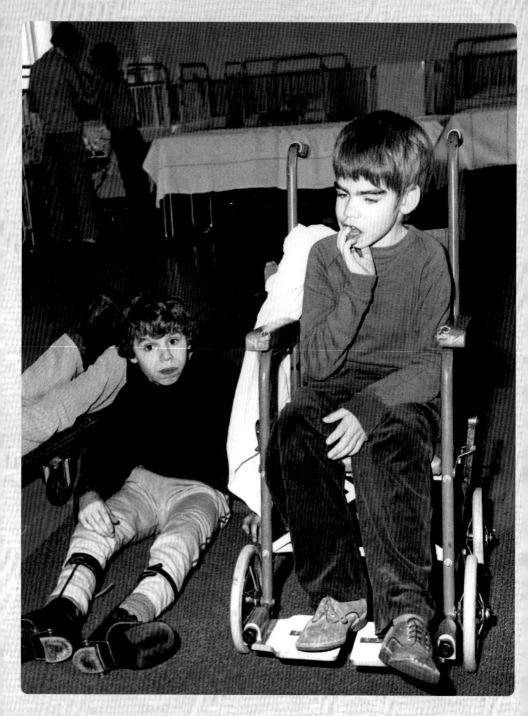

Two young residents in their ward,
circa 1975. (Courtesy of Kew Cottages
Historical Society)

up in the Penang General Hospital. At that stage nobody could work out what was causing the seizures ... About the only thing they could tell us was they didn't think it was anything hereditary. They were looking for maybe a tropical disease of some sort. During the 1980s the Children's Cottages started employing neurologists and we struck a decent, really nice neurologist and he had certain tests done on Paul ... We now believe that he suffered very serious brain damage ... [as a result of] the triple antigen injections.[46]

In August 1964, Bill and his wife Joan returned to Australia. Paul continued to experience regular seizures and was often hospitalised at the Children's Hospital where he was diagnosed with Lennox-Gastaut syndrome, a severe form of epilepsy. Bill recalled that the seizures were 'almost violent. You had to lay him down and he would kick, he was completely out of it but his limbs were still moving, arms and legs would go all over the place.'[47] Bill and Joan were traumatised watching their child endure such episodes.

Paul was the youngest of four children and while he required a lot of direct care, this did not often cause friction within the family. In fact, his brothers and sister were fiercely protective of their little brother: 'If anyone said that they had a "mad brother" ... they generally got in trouble for it.'[48] Fear of the unknown often caused such antagonism. In the 1960s, and still today, people with intellectual disability are treated with apprehension by some people in Australian society. Bill recalled that grown adults sometimes feared Paul:

Some women were a bit frightened of him. I mean he couldn't walk, but in those days he could sit on the floor and he could sort of wobble around the place and people didn't like him wobbling over near them ... and he'd touch people on the legs, too, and that sort of thing ... generally we, and he, were well accepted, but there were some people who, I'm sure, were frightened of him. I don't know why they'd be frightened of a little fella like that.[49]

The fear and apprehension expressed by some people towards children with disabilities resulted in parents often feeling stigmatised. It was hard enough to meet the emotional and everyday requirements of the immediate family, let alone spend time convincing others of the need for understanding and tolerance.

Paul's demanding medical needs and the lack of support services took their toll on the quality of life enjoyed by the Westgarth family. As Bill recalled:

> Most of those rotten seizures used to start at some ungodly hour in the morning. We weren't in the Ambulance Service at that stage. Any time we used an ambulance we had to pay for it and they wouldn't accept Paul because he had a pre-existing illness. The reason we weren't in the Ambulance Service was that we lived overseas [as I was on Australian military service] and when we came back he had the illness anyway, so we couldn't [get him cover] ... every, two, three or four weeks, we'd get him in the car and race him into the hospital into the emergency section and from there he'd always be admitted for another two or three weeks.[50]

Ferrying Paul in and out of the Children's Hospital was almost routine for the Westgarth family. Eventually a neurologist at the Children's Hospital advised them to place Paul at Kew Cottages. The neurologist believed that Kew offered Paul the necessary specialist care he required. Before placing Paul at Kew, Bill and Joan visited the Cottages. Matron Millie Lucas showed them around and they were grateful for her attention, referring to her as a 'lovely person' and a 'great help'.[51] At the age of five, in 1968, Paul was admitted to Ward 24. In 2003 he moved out of Kew and into a community residential unit located near his parents.

Who is to blame? What is to blame? These are questions that many parents of children with intellectual disability desperately seek to answer. Sometimes, however, there is no immediate explanation. This was the case for Rose and Martin Miller and their son, Sean. Rose explained: 'we really don't know what happened ... He was born perfectly normal ... [When he was] about a year old ... He just stopped developing like a baby does. He was tested for all sorts of things and nothing showed up.'[52] The local doctor referred Rose to a paediatrician who coldly told her that Sean would not develop any further. Unhappy with this doctor's attitude and prognosis, she sought a second opinion and was sent to Elizabeth Turner at the Children's Hospital. Sean underwent a battery of tests including those to determine if he had encephalitis, phenylketonuria or deafness. All tests were negative. Without a definitive diagnosis, and with the behaviours Sean was exhibiting, autism appeared a possibility.

Rose and Martin looked after Sean at home along with his brother and sister, but his challenging behaviours made life tough. Rose recalled:

> It was very frustrating … He didn't sleep. I mean you were awake all night … We had some terrible experiences. He nearly broke the house up, banging his head and that sort of thing … We had a couple of very bad experiences where somebody left the gate open and he got away. Once he got up onto [a busy, main road] … and a man carried him back. I didn't know! It turned out to be that somebody had come to the wrong house and left the gate open and he got out.[53]

The only respite the Miller family received was when the Spastic Society looked after Sean and the family went away on a two-week vacation. For Rose and Martin this break highlighted the negative effects of looking after Sean at home. Family life was suffering. The attention they gave Sean was at the expense of their other children. Rose stated that they reluctantly decided to place five-year-old Sean on the waiting list for Kew, 'I think that [it] finally got to everybody … as my sister-in-law said, "You've got to think of the greatest good for the greatest number".'[54] It took four tiring and often despairing years, but at the age of nine Sean moved to the Cottages.

It was not unusual for parents to endure lengthy waiting periods before their children's admission to Kew. For most of its history there was a constant demand for places at the Cottages. This need mostly stemmed from a lack of adequate government and community support for families who were looking after children with disabilities at home.

Although many parents believe that it was ultimately beneficial to send their children to Kew, a great many live with an enduring sense of guilt and shame at being unable to care for their sons or daughters. Parents' grief is often reflected in their faces when they speak about 'giving up' their children. Tears of sorrow and pain trickled down Hilda Logan's cheeks when she declared 'You never, ever get over it – ever.'[55] Although life had become almost unbearable for many people when they decided to commit their children to Kew, looking after their son or daughter at home had become a major part of their everyday life. Rose Miller recalled, 'I remember the day after, walking around in a circle sort of wondering: "What am I going to do?" [Sean] had absorbed the whole day. I was devastated.'[56]

For thousands of parents the road to Kew Cottages, whether chosen on a child's day of birth or years later, was a journey of great turmoil and sorrow. Medical experts were often welcome travelling companions as they offered support and guidance. However some made the experience more traumatic through a lack of understanding or empathy. Although guided by medical opinion, most parents felt responsible for their children's committal into State care. During its 121-year history the outpouring of parents' grief over the loss of their children has brought forth a river of tears.

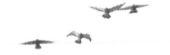

Welcome Strangers

Who is this man?
He stands alone.
Waiting.
He comes here regularly.
Collecting.

Securely wrapped in a long coat and donning a hat, he
* is fighting to stave off the icy chill of a winter seaside*
* breeze.*
Why does he look so anxiously at the ship in dock?
Who is he looking for?

He is surrounded by a bustling crowd.
These people too are staring at the mighty ship,
* anticipating the disembarkation of passengers.*

They have all come to greet someone.
Many will be reunited with relatives who have travelled
* great distances.*
Others will passionately embrace lovers kept away by
* the vast oceans.*
A few wait for work colleagues who have come to
* Australia to fill a labour shortage.*
So who is the man in the long coat and hat waiting for?

He scans the faces of a bewildered and excited line of
   passengers who march ever forward.
He is not searching for a particular person, a friend or
   relative, all before him are strangers.

The man is Dr Wilfrid Brady, the superintendent of Kew
   Cottages.
He is often seen awaiting passenger ships at Station
   Pier.
Wilfrid Brady is desperate for workers.
With the arrival of each vessel comes the hope that
   he will recruit suitable people prepared to face the
   challenge of working at Kew Cottages.
Corinne Manning, 2006

Throughout its history Kew Cottages struggled to find employees who were willing to work, often in extremely poor conditions, with people with disabilities. The inability of administrators to attract workers mostly stemmed from the widely held view that institutions such as Kew were unsavoury, depressing places where neglected, 'weird' and 'barely human' people were locked away for 'society's protection'. Media reports, which were powerful in shaping people's opinions, often constructed vivid and frightening images of Kew Cottages and its residents. For example, in 1975, an article entitled 'The Village of the Damned', published in *The Age* newspaper, described life at Kew as chaotic and volatile.[1] The article was written to encourage people to donate money to a public appeal aimed at improving facilities and services at the Cottages. In this article, residents were referred to as 'A colony of barely trained seals', 'badly worn clusters of chickens around an incubator' and 'sons and daughters of Frankenstein's monster'.[2] Even the title evoked a sense of terror, playing on the 1960 horror movie about the birth of destructive and amoral 'alien' children on Earth.[3] The language used to describe the residents was dehumanising and reflected negative stereotypes of people with intellectual disability. Throughout the 20th century, media reports created a poor image of Kew Cottages. As Wilfrid Brady waited at the docks he was hoping to attract people who had not been exposed to such disturbing reports; migrants seeking employment in their newly adopted homeland.

In addition to Kew's poor reputation, favourable economic conditions in Australia made recruitment of local workers virtually impossible at times. In the post-World War II era, Australia's economy accelerated at a breakneck pace and job opportunities were abundant. A general labour shortage resulted in higher wages and employment conditions being demanded by workers. The Cottages' management was unable to effectively compete with industries that offered employees far greater pay and better employment conditions than they could provide. In an effort to meet growing labour demands the Commonwealth Government established immigration programs to attract workers. Australia had previously engaged in assisted passage schemes, but none matched the sheer volume of immigrants who came to Australia in this era.[4] Wilfrid went to Station Pier in Port Melbourne in order to take advantage of this influx of migrant labour. It is unknown exactly what recruitment methods he used. Wilfrid may have held a placard, directly approached passengers or used existing employment agencies located at the port. Whatever means he employed, his efforts, and the direct recruitment of labour by the Australian Government, resulted in a large migrant workforce at Kew Cottages.

Sylvia Babic, who worked at the Cottages for 33 years, began her journey to Kew in 1951 when she answered an advertisement inviting British citizens to migrate to Australia. At that time, Sylvia and her friend Betty were working in Craighouse, a psychiatric hospital in Edinburgh, as ward assistants. Craving excitement and adventure, the pair applied to come to Australia as part of the £10 assisted passage scheme. Sylvia wrote:

> Betty and I were always thinking about going overseas. It didn't matter much where, so long as it was overseas. We followed up an ad in the newspaper, filled out some forms, then we had a medical … there was a shortage of staff in mental hospitals, [so we signed] … up to be student nurses in a mental hospital.[5]

At 20 years of age, they boarded the SS *Mooltan* at Tilbury Docks bound for Australia. On arrival in Melbourne, Sylvia was met by Matron Evans who drove her to her new workplace: Royal Park Mental Hospital. During her first 18 months in Australia, Sylvia worked at Royal Park, at Marlborough House in Portsea, and married a fellow migrant, a Croatian man named Charlie Babic. Unable to secure their own place, Sylvia and Charlie lived in a shared house in Kew. Charlie worked at Kew Mental Hospital and a fellow housemate worked at the Cottages. In search of work, and on the advice of her housemate, Sylvia approached the management at Kew Cottages for a job. She was successful in her efforts and commenced employment in February 1953.[6]

Although Sylvia had previously worked in institutional settings she recalled that her first day at the Cottages was taxing:

> I will never forget my first day – it was a busy one, as I carried out the duties as informed, bathing, dressing, helping at mealtimes, then looking after the children in the day room. Here I was kept very busy … It was not the best of days as my lack of practice was very visible. The other staff spoke mainly German, so it was hard to communicate.[7]

Feeling out of her depth Sylvia was reluctant to return the next day, but was convinced by her husband to stay until she received her first pay. Sylvia went back and gradually acclimatised to the world of Kew.

Kurt Kraushofer, an Austrian man, was also a £10 migrant who came to Australia in 1958. He stated that he was lured to Australia by migration advertising that promised a life of sunshine and comfort, 'I went into the Australian Embassy, saw photos and it says "300 days of sunshine". I thought that's me. I came to Australia on the 23rd of August and have never been so cold in my life!'[8] After working in a steel factory at Port Kembla and on the Snowy Mountains Scheme, Kurt moved to Melbourne where he met his wife-to-be, Maria. She was already working in Kew and organised a job for Kurt. He explained, 'I met a woman and she worked there and she's now my wife for the last 40 years. She brought me to the Cottages and my language was very limited, but somehow with her connections, I got the job and started work there.[9] Kurt never anticipated that he would spend the remainder of his working life at the Cottages.

Unlike Sylvia and Kurt, who chose to work at Kew, other migrants were assigned their positions by government authorities. These migrants were members of the 170 000 'displaced people' from Europe who entered Australia between 1947 and 1953. Their passage was paid for by the International Refugee Organization with the understanding that Australian authorities could place them in areas of employment that were essential to post-war reconstruction.[10] Some of these refugees were immediately sent to work at Kew to fill staffing shortages.[11] Other displaced people came to the Cottages after working in positions elsewhere. One such person, Maria Kraushofer, was granted a refugee visa to enter Australia and found her way to Kew. Maria was originally from Croatia and dreamt of starting a new life in this country:

> I came to Australia and lived in Albury for nine months with my sister. I decided that it's too small so I needed to go into the city. I came to Melbourne and I had friends here who already worked in [the] Cottages and I was looking for a job, so I got a job in the Cottages.[12]

Many immigrants, such as Maria, came to work at Kew through recommendations or suggestions made by people in the close-knit European migrant network that existed in Melbourne.

From the late 1960s, the migrant community at Kew evolved, as increasing numbers of people from the Asia–Pacific and African regions were employed. Once again, some of these workers came to Australia after answering job advertisements for health workers, published in overseas newspapers and journals. This was the case in regards to Saral Nathaniel, an occupational therapist (OT) from India:

> I came to know that in Australia there was …[a] shortage of physios, OTs everywhere … I said: 'Oh why shouldn't I apply and see?' I sent

a hand-written application ... to the Immigration ... I just thought: 'Oh well, there's no harm in trying.' I showed the book to Mum and Dad, they did not agree [with me]. They had a big fight ... but my brother and sister they backed me up. In India it's a very serious thing, to send your daughter [away]: 'Oh! You're not sending your daughter', 'She is not married' ... it's not only family and friends it's the neighbours too ... 'She's not going, you're not sending her to Timbuktu?' [laugh][13]

Saral was determined to prove to her family that she could survive outside of her community. She came to Australia in 1976. Initially, she accepted a position to work in Adelaide, but after six months she relocated to Melbourne. Saral moved into a house across the road from the Cottages with an Australian woman she had met in India. On the suggestion of her friend, Saral approached the Cottages and was successful in obtaining an OT position. In her mind this job was only a temporary stopover before moving into a preferred field of specialisation. She stated, 'Mental health was the *last* place I wanted to work!' Aside from a couple of extended holidays, Saral worked at Kew for 30 years.

Political and social changes in Asia resulted in many migrants and refugees coming to Australia. Dr Ruth Anghie and her family migrated to Australia from Ceylon (Sri Lanka) in 1971 because of political changes that impacted on her family's wellbeing. She explained:

My parents had been educated by English missionaries, both of them, and we were brought up in a very Western way. We appreciated everything that was Western; music, literature, everything. So when Ceylon became independent and ultra nationalist, I felt like a foreigner, I just felt I didn't belong ... for people like us who were of mixed parentage and Christian, there was absolutely no future for our children or us. We had to leave.[14]

Ruth and her husband, Trevor, who was also a medical practitioner, previously applied to come to Australia, but were denied entry because of Australia's restrictive immigration policies. Ruth recalled that when they applied again, Australian authorities were swift in approving their application:

> Within less than a week of putting our papers in we were called for an interview … George Drew was the secretary who interviewed us, and he just said: 'Oh, both of you are doctors I see, well you won't have any trouble, we need doctors', and that was it.[15]

Knowing very little about Australia, Ruth and Trevor relied on the advice of friends as to employment options. They were told that there was a need for doctors in the area of mental health. Trevor contacted the Mental Health Authority about available positions and was hired to work at Beechworth Mental Hospital.

Ruth and Trevor arrived in Australia on 27 January 1971. Ruth, who had four children, did not anticipate working as she wanted to stay at home and look after her family. However the desperate need for professional medical staff at Beechworth led to her accepting a part-time position. Although her previous experience had been largely in other medical fields, Ruth was willing to diversify her skills by working in mental health. Two years after their arrival in Australia, Ruth and her family moved to Melbourne when Trevor was given the chance to work in general practice. Ruth requested a transfer from Beechworth to Kew as she wanted to extend her experience and work among children with intellectual disability.[16] Her journey to Kew was the result of migration and a newfound interest in the mental health and disability sectors.

The paths taken to Kew Cottages by Australian workers were similar to migrants; through direct recruitment, word-of-mouth recommendation and chance. Helen Wilson was a teenager when she decided to train as a nurse and work in disability. Originally she wanted to enrol in a teaching course, but was unable to afford the tuition and living costs associated with tertiary study. Helen actively sought alternate career paths to fulfil her needs:

> I saw an ad at the back of one of my sister's nursing books … it looked so sweet. There was a picture of one person sitting on a chair with a small child, teaching, and it said: 'Have a career in intellectual disability', I think 'mental retardation' they called it back then. So I started to make some inquiries into that. I … found St Nicholas and the Children's Cottages and applied. It wasn't quite as sweet as the ad said … I was in for a big shock.[17]

In November 1972, Helen and her mother travelled to Melbourne, from Tocumwal, New South Wales, for a preliminary interview. They were met by Matron Millie Lucas who explained that Helen would receive three years practical and theoretical training by working at the Cottages and attending the onsite School of Nursing. This employment opportunity was appealing to Helen. She was immediately offered a position, but asked for a postponement in order to complete her Higher School Certificate exams. Her request was granted.

Helen returned to Kew Cottages in March 1973.[18] She was nervous about moving to Melbourne, but never considered reneging on her agreement:

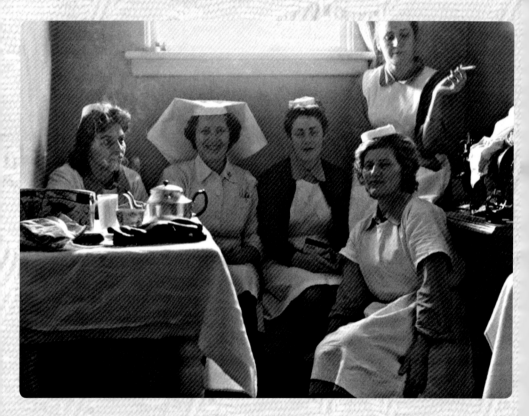

Nursing staff from Ward 38/39 taking a break in the Nurses' Room, 1961. (Courtesy of Kew Cottages Historical Society)

Back in those days when I was a teenager, we didn't have after school jobs the way the kids do these days, so it was going to be a whole new experience. Coming from a very small country town of 1000 people to Melbourne, it was very daunting … I was the youngest in the family; I didn't want to leave Mum and Dad.[19]

Helen was determined to gain professional training and forge a life of her own in the world of Kew Cottages. She succeeded and stayed at Kew until its closure.

Many medical practitioners chose to work at the Cottages in order to improve the quality of life for people less fortunate than themselves. Others combined this ideal with the practical advantages offered by the institution to conduct research into intellectual disability. In 1959, Dr David Pitt joined the Kew Cottages workforce, 'I was a paediatrician there for 17 years, and was sent there for two jobs: to improve the wretched health of the 900 children and adults, and to do research.'[20] David explained that his journey to the Cottages commenced shortly after World War II:

I was in private practice for 10 years. General practice at first which grew quickly and was lucrative, then in Collins Street for two years which was not as lucrative. So I was looking around for something to do … this offer came up through Professor Vernon Collins, at the Children's Hospital. They were looking for a full-time paediatrician at the Children's Cottages, the first one. I said: 'Oh that sounds interesting.' So I went out and had a look. I saw there were vast opportunities there for good work, original work. After negotiating for a secretary and a laboratory assistant I took the job.[21]

David was knowledgeable about Kew Cottages as he spent most of his childhood living in the Kew area. He recalled that as a boy he used to peer over the fence at 'the poor unhappy children and adults who were living under very wretched conditions'.[22] David also remembered that community attitudes were not sympathetic towards those who lived at the institution, 'Everybody feared and hated it. It was a loony-bin.'[23] David's previous contact with the Cottages and his active research interest into the causes of birth defects meant that a position at Kew was very appealing. The Cottages enabled him to contribute to the day-to-day care of disadvantaged people in the

Australian community while providing readily available subjects and facilities to continue his research. David left Kew in 1976.

Professor Malcolm Macmillan also wanted to work at Kew Cottages in order to provide residents whom he considered to be neglected with appropriate support. Malcolm was an experienced psychologist who had worked in the field of mental health and intellectual disability. In 1955, he commenced work at Travancore, the central ascertainment clinic for intellectual disability in Victoria. Through his work at Travancore, Malcolm realised that the needs of a large group of people with intellectual disability were not being met by existing programs:

> I had gradually come around to thinking that it would be a good idea if a psychologist could go to Kew to deal with the less educable kids there, the situation in the State seemed to me to be reasonably good for educable intellectually disabled people, but it was these other kids who were being left for dead and they were mostly over at Kew Cottages ... I made inquiries about going over there.[24]

Fortuitously, Malcolm's inquiries coincided with a decision by the Mental Health Authority to employ a psychologist at Kew. From 1960–64, he was employed as the Cottages' first psychologist.

While some employees sought work at the Cottages, others looked upon it as a convenient road stop where money could be made or time spent before continuing on to another destination. Michael Glenister commenced work at Kew Cottages in 1986. He had grown up in the suburb of Kew and was familiar with the institution and its residents. After leaving school, Michael was at a crossroad. Unsure of what future path to follow, he decided to apply for a job at Kew. His decision to work at Kew was primarily in order to earn money. He stated that it was:

> A means to an end. Once I actually got in the door, there were options available for courses of study and career paths. I was laughing at the time because I didn't assume that I would ever take up the options, I would just work there for a few months. At that stage I had a goal to ... purchase a motorbike and that was it, then I'd be gone.[25]

Michael's attitude was not unusual. Many workers over the years considered their employment at the Cottages to be temporary. Little did they know that on entering Kew some of them would stay for the remainder of their working lives or until its closure. Michael worked at Kew for 20 years and relocated to a community residential unit, along with a group of Kew residents, as part of the Cottages' closure and redevelopment program.

Alma Adams anticipated that her involvement at Kew Cottages would also be short-term. Originally from the United Kingdom, Alma and her family came to Australia as temporary residents when her husband was offered a contract research position. A few months after their arrival, Alma answered a job advertisement to work at Kew:

> I saw an advert in the weekend paper for coordinator of volunteers at Kew ... I know how important it is in disability to have people who are not paid staff, who have a connection with people. So I started here in '82. One of the interesting things at that time was that I had applied for what I thought was a fairly low-level job in the organisation, and it was in terms of the money that they were paying! [laugh] I was interviewed by a senior bureaucrat, Don Crawford, who was director of institutional services ... Dale Hassam, who was the new CEO of Kew, Max Jackson, who was co-ordinator of Programs, and Fran van Brummelen who was the social worker. I thought: 'My God, for a very low-level job, why am I facing a panel like this?'... Subsequently, I remember Dale telling me that it was because they felt that they were really looking to have some significant change at Kew ... I worked here until late '86, and had a short stint in '89 when Max Jackson was on leave and there was a strike on. I was asked to come back and resolve that. In December 2000, I came back with the aim of getting the redevelopment up. I came back as the manager of Kew Residential Services.[26]

Alma's latest journey to Kew has proven to be an emotional and confronting challenge as she oversees its closure. On the one hand, many people celebrate Kew's closure as a sign of social advancement as residents are incorporated into mainstream Australian society. Others consider its demise to be evidence of economic rationalism at the expense of residents' quality of life.[27]

Alongside paid employees, vast numbers of volunteer workers also journeyed to Kew. Most of these volunteers were involved with the Cottages from the post-World War II era. The reasons for people volunteering to work at Kew varied. Some were parents or relatives of residents, but a great number were strangers who wanted to contribute their spare time to improving the lives of disadvantaged people in Australian society.

Many volunteers responded to advertisements seeking support for the Cottages or media reports that described the deprivations suffered by its residents. Val Smorgon answered an advertisement calling for volunteers that was published in *The Sun* newspaper:

> I started [at Kew] because my youngest of four started …
> kindergarten that year, and I thought: 'What am I going to do?'
> Lunches are not my thing and I didn't play much sport. I happened
> to see … an ad for volunteers for Kew Cottages. I had no idea what
> Kew Cottages were, in those days people didn't really talk about
> mental retardation, it was something you didn't discuss. At school
> we never heard about it. So I saw this ad … they were looking for
> volunteers to do this training course. I think it was a ten-week
> training course … but I was leaving for overseas after three weeks,
> so I didn't finish the course. When I came back I contacted them …
> the lady that was running it … suggested that I come and help her,
> which I did. The next week she decided to leave, but I think she was
> just looking for somebody to take her place and it was me, which
> was really good because I was looking for something to do. I didn't
> actually want to be a volunteer as such, I wanted to do something
> a bit more administratively, and it turned out that that was what I
> did.[28]

For nearly ten years Val worked as the coordinator of volunteers at Kew. She was responsible for the recruitment and management of a large volunteer group, which numbered over 500 people. It was an enormous undertaking. Her initial intention of volunteering for one day a week soon ballooned into a five-day commitment. Quite unexpectedly, Val's work at Kew provided her with the opportunity to develop personally and professionally. She became one of the leading figures in Kew's history through her dedication to the Volunteer Program and her fundraising efforts for the Minus Children Appeal.

On commencing her journey to Kew she never envisaged that she would refer to it in later years as 'the best time in my life'.[29]

The journey to Kew Cottages was often a defining experience for many workers. A great many people were transient visitors lured to the Cottages by job opportunities and stable employment. Other people purposefully sought employment at the institution and devoted years, even decades, to the care and support of residents with intellectual disability. Whatever the reason, travelling along the road to Kew was only the beginning. Arriving at the destination involved a further journey into a world of pleasure and pain, hope and despair, humanity and cruelty.

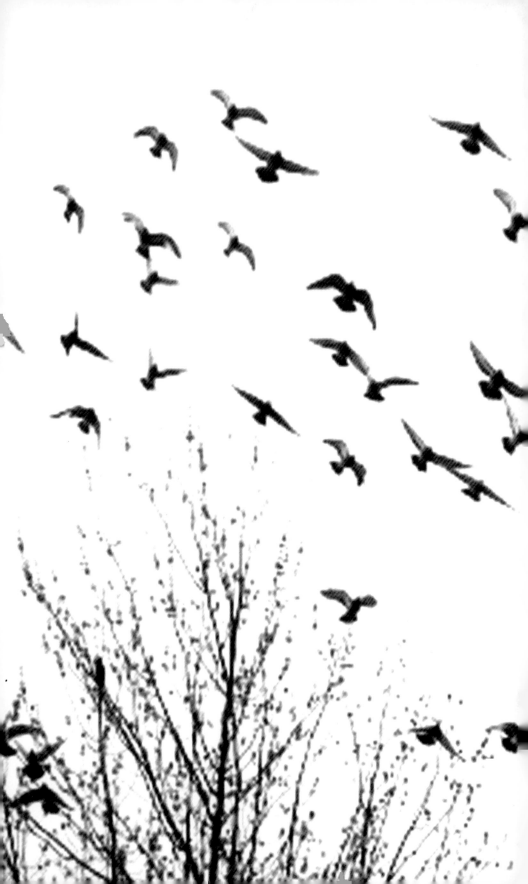

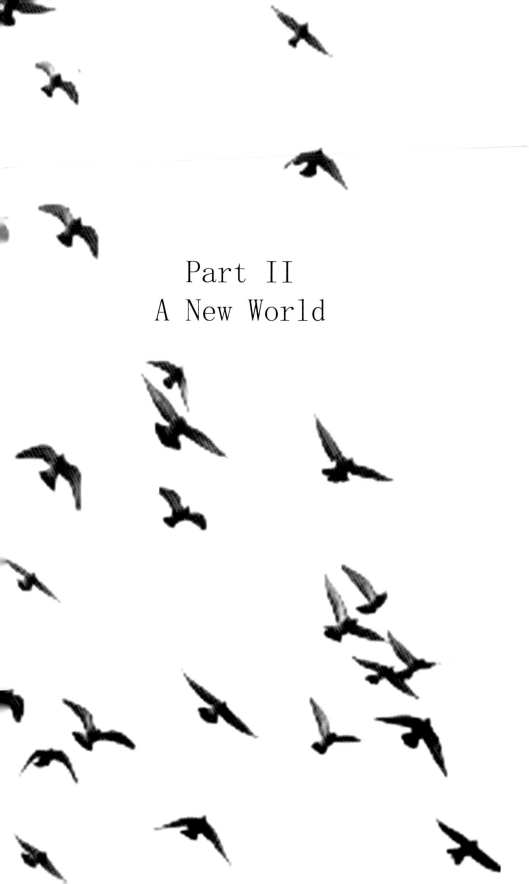

Part II
A New World

I would have loved her just to pass away as a beautiful little girl, but anyhow it wasn't to be. It brought me to a new world, out to Kew.

Anna Davison, Kew parent, 15 March 2006

On an icy winter's afternoon in 2006, I drove into the grounds of Kew Cottages. Rain began to gently patter on the windscreen as I entered through the main gate off Princess Street. Dark clouds gathered overhead, threatening a sudden downpour. I veered off to the left, driving along Main Drive, as the more direct route to my destination through Lower Drive was now closed due to the redevelopment. Over preceding months, tall, wire fences were erected cordoning off areas where residents, staff and visitors were no longer allowed to go. Within the enclosed areas skeletal forms of houses rose from the earth; the embryonic stages of a new, affluent modern suburb. Driving along, this road always feels endless as the speed limit is 20 kilometres per hour; a safety measure introduced after a resident was killed by a car. Carefully positioned, mountainous speed humps force drivers to slow down. I did not mind driving at a leisurely pace as it allowed me to survey the gardens and trees that lined the road. The English oaks and pine trees were glorious remnants of attempts by 19th-century institutional planners to beautify the landscape. They succeeded in creating stunning parkland which over the decades has become increasingly scarred through the construction of an eclectic collection of buildings commonly known as 'Kew Cottages'.

That Saturday afternoon, I was scheduled to interview a resident who had lived at Kew for 38 years. He was admitted to the Cottages at the age of six and now lived in a building known as O'Shea, a unit designed to mimic residential units available in the general community. As I drove along the road, the Cottages appeared to be well signposted. Poles scattered throughout the institution had arrows pointing to various destinations; giving a false impression of easy navigation. Due to the impending closure of the institution, many of the signed places were no longer operational and some even demolished. I studiously followed the arrows and came to a dead end. Where to from here? I knew that I had come the right way, the signpost told me so, but as I scanned the buildings I could not find O'Shea. The place was deserted! I stepped out of the car with several bags of oral history equipment. Right on cue the heavens opened up. Resembling a pack-horse, I madly dashed towards the familiar metal walkway that winds its way around the institution. I looked up, salvation! A white mini-bus was headed towards me; help was on its way.

When the bus stopped two residents alighted and approached me. The first man was tightly wrapped in a parka with buttons fastened up to his neck. He was wearing a thick woollen hat, scarf and gloves. His eyes were magnified by a pair of oval shaped, thick spectacles that highlighted his deep, chocolate brown eyes. He had obviously just come back from shopping as he clutched a bag in his hand. The outline of a toy blue car pressed against the wet, translucent plastic:

CORINNE Excuse me, I was wondering if you could help me? I'm lost and can't find my way to O'Shea. Could you please show me where it is?

DONALD It's over there.

He was pointing to a building directly in front of us. As we walked towards the doorway I extended my hand and introduced myself: 'Hi, I'm Corinne.' He shook my hand and replied:

DONALD I'm Donald.

CORINNE Are you Donald Starick?

DONALD Yeah.

CORINNE I've come to interview you today.

As he turned and smiled, I noticed that the second resident was walking close behind us. Introductions were exchanged: Raymond Bouker, another future participant in the history project. On this freezing afternoon, in an institution that housed approximately 100 residents supported by direct care staff, it seemed extraordinary that Donald and I should meet this way.

As we headed for O'Shea, I thought how fortuitous that meeting was, but the adage 'if you want to find your way around an institution just ask a resident' also sprang to mind. During my research for this project there were many times when I relied upon residents to navigate me around the Cottages. Kew's expansive grounds and maze-like arrangement were constantly challenging. Although some residents were able to verbally communicate, others used sign language or took my hand and led to me to the requested destination. It was not surprising that residents were so knowledgeable about Kew Cottages, as many of them spent decades living within its confines.

In order to understand the daily world of Kew I have chosen to focus upon issues that were important to residents and their experience of living in an institution. The following chapters discuss some of the major issues raised by residents in our conversations and recorded oral histories. A range of oral testimony has been included in every chapter to reflect institutional life and the relationships formed between various people, most notably residents, staff, family and volunteers. An understanding of the complex nature of life at Kew emerges through exploring subjects such as personal care, food, clothing, education, work, relationships and safety. Through peoples' memories I discovered that in fact many worlds existed within the institution.

CHAPTER 3

Beyond
'Fairyland'

*This little area has a special place in my
heart ... what we see here, we used to call
when we were young 'Fairyland', because for
kids it was red mushrooms and toadstools,
and heaps of wildflowers ... in our childhood
we were always coming down here on our
bikes and playing cowboys and Indians.*

Philip Brady, son of the superintendent,
Wilfrid Brady, 9 November 2006

Philip Brady's memories of life at Kew Cottages are happy
reminiscences filtered through the eyes of a child. On 9 November
2006, Philip took me on a Kew Cottages walking tour highlighting
places of personal significance. His father was a psychiatrist, Dr
Wilfrid Brady, who worked in both the Cottages and the Mental
Hospital from the 1930s, and rose to the rank of superintendent of
Kew Cottages in 1958. Philip's parents lived in a government-owned
home, situated in Wills Street, which ran adjacent to the Cottages.
According to family legend, his mother was seen clambering over the
hillside between the Hospital and Cottages picking wildflowers the
day before he was born. As we stood in that exact location surveying

the bush landscape, Philip evoked images of childhood antics and bygone days. His relationship with the Cottages and its inhabitants was one of privilege. Philip and his childhood friends were able to freely explore the grounds, creating imagined worlds and enjoying the parkland that enveloped both institutions. For Philip, it was an extraordinary place of wonderment. However, for most residents at the Cottages the physical landscape was oppressive.

The provision of government housing for some employees at Kew Cottages meant that their personal and working lives were often spent within the bounds of the institution. Increasingly, from the 1950s, many people who worked at Kew bought or rented houses away from the Cottages. This was due to the limited availability of staff housing. Those eligible for staff accommodation included high-ranking doctors and their families and selected workers, most notably single, female nurses. Employees, such as the superintendent, were allocated residences on the periphery of the institution in Wills Street. Although staff accommodation was convenient, the location meant that complete separation of work and home life was impossible. Philip Brady's sister, Jeannette Hodgkinson, highlighted the physical connection of her home to the institution, 'We had an old fashioned telephone on the wall just for the Cottages.'[1] She claimed that her father would be on call 24 hours a day.

Many staff and their relatives became accustomed to living in close proximity to the institution and used its facilities and open spaces for recreational purposes. Philip and Jeannette recalled that Sundays were a time for social tennis, when employees and their families would congregate around the Cottages' tennis court, 'it was always very social on a Sunday afternoon for all the doctors and their wives to come up here and play tennis. We used to have a little grandstand ... it was sort of like a mini Kooyong.'[2] During this era, in the 1940s and '50s, most residents watched people wandering past and enjoying the Cottages' grounds from behind a wire fence. Jeannette wrote, 'My sister, Diane and I would often play tennis on a court in the grounds – there was a large area outside with a high fence all around it – male patients, in heavy Army coats

Living in the Nurses' Home

In the early 1970s, Helen Wilson lived in the onsite Nurses' Home at Kew Cottages. She recalled the fear that 'matron's inspections' evoked, 'if there was ever an inspection at the Nurses' Home you'd always see all of these burgundy capes flying across the grounds because they'd been warned that matron was coming to do a check on the rooms. So you had to rush back there to make sure your room was tidy because you'd get into trouble if it wasn't.'

(Interview with Helen Wilson, 8 March 2006)

... would continually pace up and down, calling out all the time – a very sad sight.'[3]

In the 1970s, trampolines were situated near many wards. These were introduced as a means of offering an activity for residents to enjoy at the Cottages. They also served as a drawcard for staff and a few locals. Nurse, Helen Wilson, recalled that when she lived in the Nurses' Home a lot of staff played on the trampolines at night. This playfulness was in contravention of institutional regulation, but was too tempting for staff living close by. Matron Millie Lucas severely reprimanded a local man for taking advantage of Kew's trampolines. According to parent Bill Westgarth:

she and I walked around the Cottages this particular day and here was a bloke trampolining his dog. Oh, didn't she give him a serve, she really, really hoed into him! ... He took it all, although he didn't get much of a choice ... I suppose you're seeing a red-veiled woman coming towards you, in a fiery mood, you're not really going to stand around with your dog. He listened to her, I don't think he said more than a couple of words, 'yes' and 'no' and went.[4]

Another incident involved a local neighbourhood boy, who broke his arm after falling off a trampoline. This accident resulted in signs being erected by Kew administration stating that the trampolines were for residents' use only. The signs were not meant to curb local interaction with the institution, but to stop litigation if an 'unauthorised' person was injured while playing on the equipment. It was not unusual for people from the local neighbourhood to use Kew's grounds as a public park. While this was tolerated to a certain extent, there was an expectation by Kew staff that visitors would respect institutional property.

While many residents observed passers-by from behind a wire barricade, a few entered this outside world. This privileged group of residents were those chosen by professional staff to attend education and training programs, or were employed in various jobs within the institution. Resident, Lois Philmore, a domestic employed in the Brady household, recollected, 'I helped Dr Brady and Mrs Brady in Kew ... in the morning ... I did all the ironing, cleaning the bath, and the housework.'[5] Other residents were uninvited guests, knocking on the front door of staff houses, or entering via backyard gates that opened onto institutional land. Astrid Judge, the daughter of psychiatrist Dr Cliff Judge, remembered being hesitant and sometimes afraid, particularly of one male resident, who sometimes came into her property without invitation:

> We didn't like the young silent nonverbal man who would open the back gate of our house and walk straight into our kitchen, where mum would be preparing dinner and have to use some force and determination to get him away from us. Sometimes he would push past and start opening cupboards in the hall, or stride down to our bedrooms. Occasionally, his head appeared at our bedroom window while we were dressing, which terrified us the most because this window was on the side of our house accessible from the street outside the Cottages, and this man was certainly not supposed to have been moving around outside the grounds of the institution.[6]

Freedom to roam was enjoyed mostly by an elite group of 'high functioning' residents who were able to navigate around Kew and

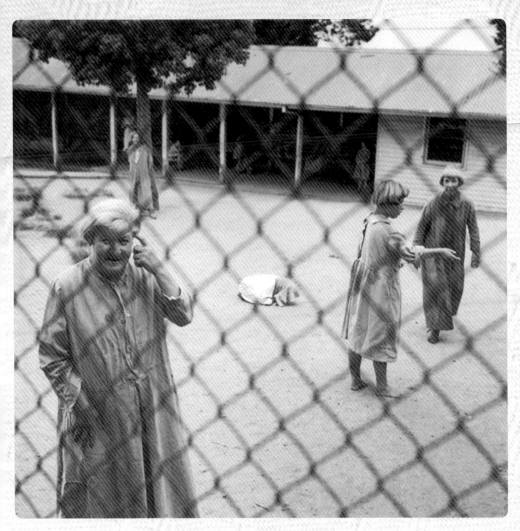

Residents in an airing court (yard) at
Kew Cottages, 1951. (Courtesy of Kew
Cottages Historical Society)

its environs unassisted by staff. A lack of direct supervision was probably why the 'nonverbal man' was able to venture into the wider suburb of Kew. This man behaved in a manner that was familiar to him, as staff and others peered into the residents' world without their permission.

Up until the 1960s, many residents spent their days outside. Although shelter sheds were provided, there was only a small fireplace to keep them warm. Ward assistant, Ted Wilson, explained that in the 1940s and '50s, 'Whether it was rain or shine in those days they all went into the airing court.'[7] The airing courts were mostly concreted yards where fences were erected to contain residents. Austra Kurzeme started work as a ward assistant in July 1953. On her first day she returned from breakfast to find that her assigned group of residents had vanished. Austra discovered that a nurse had locked them outside so that she could complete cleaning duties without interruption, 'I found them in the yard ... locked in like a big cage ... without a roof.'[8] Austra explained that there was little to keep residents entertained:

> There was one big wheel that they used, they were sitting for hours on end, going round there, and some were playing with a little grass, you know, take one blade of grass and sit in the corner and nod, and about 10 or 15 of them were busy untying the laces and pulling the buttons off, and undressing.[9]

By restricting residents' movement within defined areas, staff were able to carry out duties inside the dormitories without the additional burden of overseeing their charges.

It was not unusual for one staff member to be stationed outside with up to 70 people. In order to prevent residents from absconding, many of these enclosures were framed by high wire fences and locked with a special key. Despite physical barriers and staff supervision, there were a few residents who absconded, enjoying stolen moments of liberty until caught and often punished. Due to his position as a 'working resident', Patrick Reed was allowed to freely roam around Kew Cottages during most of his stay at the institution. Initially, Patrick was locked indoors and in airing courts with fellow residents. He was incredibly bored being shut away and tried to escape with others, 'Oh, it was boring ... Just walking around, the whole yard was full of kids ... that's why we nicked off.'[10] Austra chased after a resident who scaled the mesh fence and ran off into institutional grounds nearby. Her enthusiasm to catch the escapee meant that 70 other residents were left unattended and she was duly reprimanded by the charge nurse. On one occasion Ted Rowe stopped a fellow resident from running away telling him of the consequences:

TED A few tried to escape, I wasn't game to escape.

CORINNE Why were they trying to escape, can you remember?

TED Because they don't like the place, that's why … One of them said to me one day, 'Oh gees I'd like to get away from here' and I said 'You won't get out because the doors are locked.' 'Oh that's bad … I'll have to do something [about that].' I said 'The only way … is don't come back in when they come to lock the door and [then] you're out there. You can do what you like. But they'll be after you … [they'll] find out where you've gone and you'll cop it then, by gee you would.' They do cop it. You could hear them yelling out, 'No, no, no!' They knew they were going get the strap on the backside.

CORINNE So did that boy sneak out?

TED He never sneaked out, no. He was too scared.[11]

However, the taste of a little freedom and the chance to get out of the institutional confines proved too tempting for some residents, even if such transgressions resulted in punishment.

While Philip Brady and his friends were playing in 'Fairyland' in the 1940s and '50s, many residents were forced to endure hours of boredom. Sylvia Babic recalled that in the 1950s many residents with high and complex support needs were frequently bedridden, trapped within the dormitory. A few of these residents and all ambulant residents were relocated each day to seats and benches on outside verandahs or in day rooms.[12] These areas were stark spaces with minimal furnishings and often no activities available for residents. To add to the boredom, during this period ward staff spent most of their time completing daily tasks to keep the ward running, rather than spending time playing, conversing or inter-

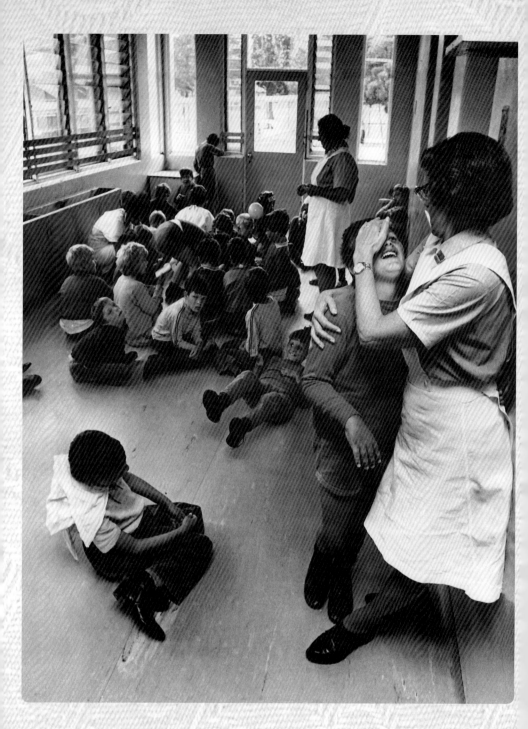

A typical day room where residents were confined, 1975. (Courtesy of *The Age* Archives/*The Age*, Melbourne)

acting with residents. Austra Kurzeme stated, 'there were so many duties you had to do ... you hardly had time to go and look at the girls'.[13] Even residents, who left the confines of the wards for periods of time were faced with boredom on return. Ralph Dawson was critical of being locked away in dormitories stating that it was 'too much boring'.[14]

Despite the occasional toy donation drive for the Cottages, there were very few toys for children to play with or equipment and activities for older children and adults. In the 1970s, Dianne Pymble was instructed to give residents paper to rip as there were no toys.[15] At times when toys were in the wards, they were sometimes kept away from residents for fear of them breaking or ruining the prized items. When the chairman of the Mental Hygiene Authority, Dr Eric Cunningham Dax, inspected the Cottages he noticed that toys in one ward were stored out of the reach of children. He immediately ordered that these be distributed as their purpose was for play, not display.[16] Outside games, although rare, were sometimes played by residents of all ages. In the 1920s and '30s, Ted Rowe enjoyed playing typical Australian sports, 'we had a good old time together and we used to play cricket or football'.[17] By the 1950s and '60s these activities do not appear to be commonplace. Patrick Reed, who came to live at Kew in 1955, had no recollection of any games or equipment available in his area during this period. After breakfast he had to 'Go in the yard.'[18] Occasionally residents were taken by staff on walks throughout the grounds or to a nearby oval to participate in outdoor sports, but up until the 1960s, these were also rare events.

For decades most residents survived within limited physical environments that often challenged the senses. Although Philip Brady's initial recollections of Kew were mostly positive, our tour of the grounds triggered forgotten memories, important features of institutional life. As we sat on a park bench next to the tennis court overlooking the Cottages, Philip declared:

> they've only just come back to me ... Two things that will remain vivid in my mind ... Day and night, as you grow up, there were

always bloodcurdling screams coming from nearby, from the different wards. I also remember the stench that used to waft across when there was a northerly wind blowing ... back in those days, 60 years ago and beyond, I imagine the sewerage left something to be desired.[19]

These sensory memories illuminated a side of institutional life that is sometimes lost through time, but highlight critical issues that greatly impacted on the lives of people working, residing and visiting Kew Cottages. If the screams were clearly audible from staff houses, imagine their volume within the wards. As Ralph Dawson testified,

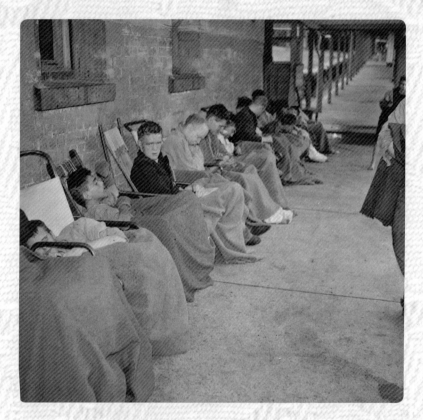

Residents outside their dormitory at Kew, 1951. Many residents were seated outside every day with little or no activities on offer. (Courtesy of Cliff Judge, private collection)

'Boys [were] screaming too much, they drive me up the wall ... [They] made too much noise, I had to block my ears.'[20] When I asked David Honner, a resident admitted in 1958, about dormitory life he agreed with Ralph:

CORINNE What was it like?

DAVID Too noisy.

CORINNE And did you ever try to get away from the noise?

DAVID Yes, but I couldn't.[21]

In the 1990s, when David Sykes was coordinator of the Citizen Advocacy Inner East Program, he visited Kew:

> even though they had their own small separate or shared rooms, the noise-level was phenomenal ... You'd go in and more often than not they'd already be in front of the TV in there, or just lying in their beds ... And even in the units that didn't have the old cavernous ceiling, the noise level was just extraordinary. Certainly we felt, with some of the residents, that their only way of dealing with that was to retreat into themselves, whether it was the foetal position stuff or on the couch rocking back and forth. We'd often leave Kew and the conversations or thinking would be: 'Oh I think I'd probably do the same thing!' In that extremely loud environment where people are screaming and the staff might be yelling out to deal with some stuff, how do you live in that environment?[22]

Staff often spoke about 'getting used' to harsh conditions, but the fact was that they could leave Kew, whereas residents were forced to continually endure these conditions hour upon hour, day after day.

The persistent overcrowding that plagued the Cottages from its earliest years contributed to excessive noise levels. From 1888, as funds for building and improvements were made available from the Victorian Government or public donation, additional facilities were erected. Major exceptions to periods of intense overcrowding were the late 1930s, when hundreds of residents were sent to live at other residential training institutions, such as Janefield, and more recently through deinstitutionalisation programs. In 1937, a Coronial Inquest concluded that overcrowding was a key contributor to the death of a 28-year-old resident, Thelma Ada Hills.[23] Thelma was fatally scalded when the nurse in charge of her ward attended to a fight that had broken out between residents. During the inquest it was revealed that the nurse was solely in charge of 44 residents. Thelma's death caused a public scandal and shone the spotlight on inadequate levels of staffing and overcrowding at the Cottages.

Throughout its history the demand for places at Kew Cottages often exceeded supply. In 1959, social worker, Irena Higgins, published the first waiting list for people requiring State care in institutions such as Kew. In 1960, 140 people were registered on Kew Cottages' waiting list.[24] In order to accommodate a maximum number of residents, beds and mattresses were crammed into wards. Margaret Cotter was working elsewhere as a nurse when she first visited Kew in the 1950s. She was disgusted by the overcrowded dormitories, 'I went there a few times and in those days they had mattresses under the beds because it was so overcrowded … I couldn't *believe* that these patients could be sleeping on mattresses underneath a bed. They got pushed back under the bed of a daytime, and pulled out for the night, that really appalled me.'[25]

Many Kew staff recognised that overcrowding resulted in substandard living conditions. A few even tried to make improvements by suggesting practical alterations to inadequate living arrangements. Jack Cotter, secretary and manager at Kew from 1971–80, stated 'Even some of the units that were reasonable, fabric-wise and [in regards to] equipment, still had problems because they had too many residents in them. These dedicated nursing staff used to come up with lots of funny schemes about how they might improve things, you know double-deck beds and all that sort of thing, but the real problem was that there were just too many bodies in them.'[26] From the 1980s deinstitutionalisation programs resulted in a small number of residents moving away from the Cottages and into community housing. Alterations in institutional structures were gradually being made to provide more private living spaces. However, in 1989, a local newspaper reported that overcrowding was still a major problem at the institution.[27]

Aside from a few public appeals, most notably Tipping (1953) and Minus Children (1975), politicians and the general public were apathetic towards Kew Cottages. Although, mainly from the late 1930s, newspaper articles about the plight of people living at Kew were published several times a year, essential resources to provide a quality standard of living for residents were rarely forthcoming. According to Alma Adams, manager of Kew in 2007, this constant battle for resources over time resulted in a kind of 'Blitz spirit' forming among staff. The creation of a staff identity centred upon the nobility of enduring hardship, meant that these conditions were normalised as an inherent part of the institutional world, and were sometimes celebrated as a badge of honour. This was significant among long serving staff who had 'sacrificed' their working lives to the institution. However, staff could flee these challenging circumstances at the end of their shift and go home to creature comforts such as a soft bed, private bathroom and relative peace. Surely if badges for 'courage' and 'determination' were to be awarded, residents should receive first honours for surviving such adversity.

Prior to the 1960s, the Cottages were segregated with separate male and female divisions, except for the nursery and young children's wards. Physical demarcations were created through the construction of fences. Residents were closely monitored by staff. Ted Wilson was forthright when discussing the vigilance of staff in regards to segregation in the 1940s and '50s, 'If a fellow went across – "Back!" If a girl went across – "Back!"'[28] Enforcement of this rule was echoed by resident Ted Rowe, who chuckled as he recalled, 'the gate was normally locked. See the girls yelled out, "Here, the gate's unlocked, come on up" so we went in and all the boys [were] running around starting to kiss the girls and that. And then anyhow this warder saw it, "Get out of there", he said. "Get back on your own side of the fence!"'[29] There were various reasons for segregation which ranged from practicalities in administrative processes to prohibiting sexual contact, not solely between residents, but also potentially staff and residents.[30] There were times when male and female residents mixed, but these were often social events or work details where staff monitored personal interaction. This surveillance emphasised the unequal power relationship that existed at the Cottages and highlighted the existence of different worlds that intersected under strict staff control. However, when opportunities arose, residents took full advantage of barriers breaking down. Ted Wilson even claimed that he knew of a couple of babies that were born as a result of sexual liaisons at Kew Cottages.[31]

Not only were residents separated according to gender, but staff as well. When the gender barrier was abolished in the 1960s, some male and female staff members were assigned to work together. Many people believed that through mixing staff a more balanced approach to care for residents would be achieved. Jack Cotter recalled some of the difficulties of eradicating gender separation. He described one occasion when a female staff member became overawed when working in a male dormitory, 'I think the sight of a bunch of these fellas in the shower one night [unsettled her], she fled screaming from the place … she was *exposed* a bit too suddenly to the naked bodies of these youths and young men and it was too much for her.'[32] Ruth Anghie spoke of the difficulties facing male staff working in the female wards:

> when they put male staff into the dependent units it was a bit difficult … For the males to have to look after totally dependent female residents, especially when they were menstruating, wasn't pleasant or easy … [I would] have to speak to the unit manager and say: 'All the bathing and the things like this, it will take a while for them to get accustomed to doing it.'[33]

By the 1970s segregation was no longer a major issue at Kew. The liberalisation of movement between the sexes did not necessarily accord with greater freedoms for residents; staff were as vigilant as ever to ensure that sexuality and sexual behaviour were kept in check.

Safety was one of the major reasons for many families placing their relatives into care at the Cottages. Parents, such as Hilda Logan, Rose Miller and Geoff and Elsie Welchman, had experienced the terror of searching for their children after they escaped from home. Kew Cottages appeared to offer a safe and controlled environment. At night time many residents were locked indoors, this was standard practice for some areas up until the late 20th century. Ted Rowe recalled that he would be marched into the dormitories and locked in at night, so that no one could escape, 'The dormitories were all in one, like brown cows, you're walking up there to get to your bed ... you stay in there till they unlock the door next morning for breakfast.'[34] In addition to night time safety, the Cottages were located next to the Yarra River and from the 1930s in close proximity to a major highway. Many staff felt that the physical safety of residents was at risk if they were allowed to walk around unsupervised.

Their concerns were not unfounded. On occasion there were stark reminders of the dangers of moving beyond the institution's bounds. Jack Cotter recounted that during his time a resident was found dead in the Yarra, having drowned after wandering away from the Cottages.[35] Kurt Kraushofer supported Jack's claims, 'We had a few incidents. You know that Kew is surrounded by the Yarra and some people went for walks and they didn't realise that they're not Jesus Christ, they couldn't walk across the Yarra and we had a couple of drownings.'[36] Kurt was also quick to point out these incidents also occurred in the general community. He believed that it was healthier for residents to take advantage of the open spaces and parkland at the Cottages, rather than being shut away. However, many institutional managers, staff and families of residents considered that an inherent part of Kew's duty of care towards residents was harm minimisation through the use of strict physical controls.

Residents who were able to walk around Kew were often involved in organised activities, such as the Special School. These people belonged to a privileged group who were considered to be 'higher functioning' and ambulant. In the early 1940s, if it was fine weather, school teacher Evelyn Richards escorted her class to nearby grasslands to let her children roll down the hills. On other days she took them for walks through the grounds, taking in the beauty of the natural environment. During one of their walks they chanced upon a woman singing:

> It was a beautiful day and the children and I stood stock still because we heard a woman patient in the main building singing beautifully. The whole thing was extraordinary, this beautiful spring day – this loud, beautiful voice soaring, I thought, to unprecedented heights. Subsequently, I found out there was a patient in the main building who had been a trained singer.[37]

In the 1950s and '60s, more residents took advantage of an increased number of therapy and kindergarten sessions. Institutional photos from this era depict 'happy' children, playing, singing and dancing. These photos reflect popular family images from this era; children building towers from a colourful assortment of wooden blocks, train tracks being carefully constructed and kids playing water games on a hot summer's day. Most of these images represent children taking part in schooling and therapy sessions; many were shot for publicity purposes. By contrast, it is rare to find photographs taken inside the wards where conditions were poor. For residents who were deemed by staff to be unsuitable for such programs, life remained mundane and secluded.

Some residents were allowed to venture beyond the institution. Many of these residents were classified 'workers' who were employed locally or were ordered by staff to complete tasks away from the institution. In the 1960s, Lois Philmore was proud of being entrusted to leave the Cottages and go to the local shops, 'Miss Lucas … let me go down the street on me own … because she trusted me … I'd do shopping for the people and staff.'[38] From the 1960s, as a result of Cunningham Dax's reforms which were aimed at opening up institutions, more residents utilised the Kew grounds and explored the surrounding suburb. Maria Kraushofer said that these reforms were not without incident as some residents were returned to the Cottages by police who falsely assumed they had 'escaped'.[39] Although some residents took advantage of this newfound liberty, many others remained in wards and airing courts psychologically locked into a routine they had experienced for decades. Kurt Kraushofer noted, 'Once we opened the doors, we had a couple of people expanding their environment, but basically they stayed there [in the unit].'[40] Perhaps the reluctance of some residents to move beyond the wards and airing courts was due to a fear of delving into unfamiliar territory. Others were reliant upon staff members to assist them as they were constrained by physical disabilities. On occasion some residents took on this staff role. For example, Nick Konstantaras recalled assisting his friend David Honner to get to the kiosk by pushing his wheelchair.[41] Many residents were able to move outside of their wards because their friends were willing to push their wheelchairs around the meandering walkways or help sight impaired residents navigate the uneven and undulating terrain.

As Kew Cottages often epitomised contemporary thinking towards intellectual disability, in the 1970s and '80s it operated according to the developmental model and normalisation principles. The developmental model advocated that people with intellectual disability had the potential to develop and learn. Normalisation purported making available, to people with intellectual disability, patterns and conditions of everyday life that resembled those found in mainstream society.[42] Four training and education centres were established to enable residents to participate in programs that reflected these ideals. Programs were designed to improve independent living skills and provide stimulating activities outside of the living accommodations. The new centres attempted to cater for as many residents as possible.

Due to institutional changes, a greater number of residents attended programs, but understaffing resulted in demand often exceeding supply. Some residents were unable to access these opportunities, or received very short program sessions. Alma Adams recalled, 'not everybody had access ... because there weren't the resources, some people only got as little as two hours a week'.[43] Despite the limited nature of programs on offer, staff member, John Wakefield witnessed improvements among residents within a matter of weeks, 'When people started to get dressed and go out of the ward every day, for at least two hours a day, all those macabre behaviours disappeared. Before that people were bored out of their mind and that was so marked.[44] This improvement appeared to be proof of the way in which the physical environment affected the behaviours and quality of life enjoyed by residents at the Cottages.

Although the nature of life at Kew had altered in the 1970s and '80s, Kew staff and residents continued to endure problems that existed previously. Many direct care staff still grappled with over-crowded units and heavy workloads. Christine Walton's brother, Michael, was a resident at Kew during this period. She noted that staff:

> were so busy doing the basics that there was very little time for frills, and it was nobody's fault, definitely no-one's fault at the operational level. So the opportunity to take time out just to stop and listen, or to talk or to caress if it was appropriate, just didn't happen because there was so much in just dealing with the physical needs and what had to be done.[45]

A lack of interpersonal interaction between staff and residents persisted under the new administration. The physical landscape of the Cottages was also little changed. Life inside the Cottages remained routine and communal.

In the 1980s and '90s, disability rights and advocacy movements encouraged greater individualisation for residents and attempted to address issues of inequity. However, within a large institution such as Kew, overcrowding and oppressive institutional practices tended to obviate such reforms. From the 1980s, efforts were made to impart a sense of individual living within the institution by partitioning dormitories into smaller, shared living spaces and creating semi-independent living accommodations, such as the Avenue Hostel, O'Shea and residential units located in perimeter houses on Wills and Princess streets. However, it was only in the 1990s that the majority of residents were able to live in this type of accommodation as previously places were strictly limited to residents who were considered to be 'higher functioning'. Administration and services remained largely centralised. The greatest change brought about by reforms in disability policies and principles was that the majority of residents were able to access work placements and/or programs. While some of these were located outside of the institution, many remained onsite as part of the Minus Children's buildings, OT Workshop, Network Q and Kew Day Programs. By the early 21st century, everyday life for many residents remained predominantly within the narrow confines of the units, facilities and grounds of Kew Cottages.

CHAPTER 4

'No Buttons, No Braces and No Laces!'

*At 6.30 every morning the asylum bells rang.
Before the radio and electric clocks those bells
were the time signal for lots of people around
the area [to awaken].*

Harry Willoughby, resident of the suburb of
Kew and Kew parent, 1987

This recollection was shared by Harry Willoughby who grew up
in a house located in Princess Street, opposite Kew Cottages, from
1916–39. While the bells of the 'main building' heralded a new day
for people in the suburb of Kew and its environs, residents remember
a more personal approach to waking at the Cottages. Ralph Dawson
recalled that in the morning, 'Someone would wake me up, [they said]
"Time to get up" and I bounced out of bed.'[1] As dormitories were
standard accommodations up until the late 20th century, at around
7 am row after row of residents were woken to commence the day's
routine. Raymond Bouker was aged five when he went to live at Kew
in 1959. He described the morning routine in his ward, 'Seven o'clock
… Get dressed and have breakfast and then brush your teeth.'[2] Ralph
and Raymond's reminiscences may appear familiar to many people

living in mainstream Australian society, however an examination of personal care at Kew reveals a highly regimented, often deprived and oppressive world. Throughout its history, life in this large institution was vastly different from Australian homes.

In State facilities such as Kew Cottages, bathing, showering and toileting were public events, watched by fellow residents and staff. Ted Rowe described the open layout of toilets in his area during the 1920s and '30s, 'They got these big lines of drums ... [with] a seat built on top of it ... and you sit down in that.'[3] The seat that Ted referred to was a long wooden bench with multiple seats cut out. Nurse, Sylvia Babic, described these toilets as still being in use in the 1950s.[4] This toilet arrangement was by no means private,

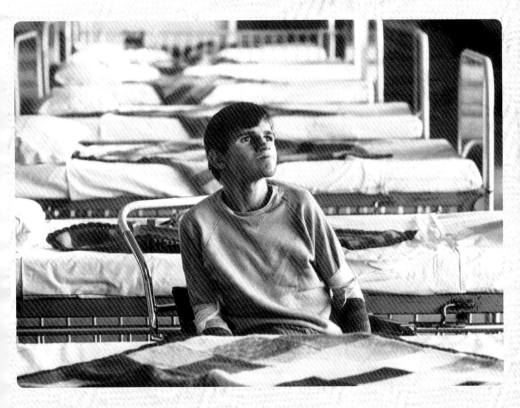

A resident in his dormitory at Kew, 1975. (Courtesy of *The Age* Archives/ *The Age*, Melbourne)

but was luxurious in comparison to the open troughs and chamber pots that were commonly used elsewhere. In 1962, John Wakefield worked in a ward located in 'Little Pell', an area of the Cottages that consisted of corrugated iron huts that were redistributed from a former Army camp after World War II. John recalled that these accommodations were some of the most deprived at Kew, 'Forty boys using one shower, which was unbelievable, and no toilets.'[5] Residents who were housed in these wards were forced to use chamber pots or an outside communal toilet block.

Even though some toileting facilities were available, up until the 1960s, everyday living conditions were sullied by urine and faeces that dirtied both the residents and their environment. Some residents were toilet trained and able to use the conveniences on offer. Many other residents received no training or needed support. With so few staff, it was often difficult to keep up with cleaning demands. In 1953, within minutes of starting her first shift at Kew, Austra Kurzeme was confronted by the reality of life at the Cottages. As she walked through the ward she noticed her charges 'huddling in a heap on the floor, cold, half naked and half of them already smeared with faeces and the smell!'[6] After bathing some residents and delivering breakfast, Austra went outside to find that nearly all of the residents were 'filthy – all incontinent … no nappies, plenty of stink and flies, and the floor full of faeces!'[7] During this period nappies were often worn by babies and toddlers. Older residents who were incontinent were often left sitting in soiled clothes, blankets, chairs and bedding. In later years cloth nappies were more frequently used for older residents.

Securing essential supplies, such as nappies, was an endless task for many staff. Although the onsite sewing room made thousands of nappies throughout the years, there were never enough to satisfy demand. Nurse, Helen Wilson, outlined one method used by some staff to obtain additional nappies for their residents:

> Laundry supplies were very short back in the '70s, so you sometimes did devious tricks. You had laundry bags numbered with your unit number on it … you'd often resort to going and pinching off another

Laundry Wars

Until the late 20th century, soiled clothes and linens were collected every day from the wards and sent to a central facility for cleaning. When staff uniforms were mandatory, these were also laundered onsite. Kew's laundry service was a constant bone of contention between laundry and ward staff. Kew manager, Jack Cotter, noted that even as late as the 1970s, 'The laundry was a great battleground really. The unit staff were always complaining about the standard of the laundry, things that were lost and [unit staff] claiming that the laundry owed them hundreds of sheets and the laundry saying: "We do not!" It was an ongoing problem.' Nurse Helen Wilson was critical of aspects of the laundry service, 'there were lots of problems with the laundry. You'd send things out and they wouldn't come back, they'd go missing.' In an effort to gain some control, a few staff and residents washed special or essential items of clothing in the units. Helen stated, 'In certain units you would do some of the better things. You did small things like the socks and the undies probably, bras for the ladies, woollen things ... if there was something really special, you'd hand wash it'. Many ward staff were puzzled and frustrated when doctors' and nurses' uniforms returned from the laundry crisp, white and neatly ironed, in contrast to the poor quality of service for residents.

(Interviews with Jack and Margaret Cotter, 6 March 2006 and Helen Wilson, 8 March 2006)

unit and putting their *dirty* nappies into your numbered bag so it'd
come back to *you*! That meant that that unit went short, but then
it was up to them to fight and try and get more. You went to some
desperate measures sometimes to make sure that your residents had
the best service.[8]

With the introduction of nappies for general use for incontinence,
residents were still often left sitting in urine and faeces as in many
cases understaffing meant that nappies were not changed immediately
after soiling. The advent of disposable undergarments for adults, in
the late 20th century, drastically improved the quality of their life.
These garments provided much greater absorbency and comfort. Staff
also benefited from this innovation as they were no longer required
to obtain, launder and fold a never-ending supply of cloth nappies.

Up until the late 1950s toilet and sewerage facilities were poor
at Kew. In the 1930s and '40s, public monies were diverted into programs to help alleviate the effects of the Great Depression and to
support World War II. As a result of these economic policies many
public institutions fell into disrepair. In the late 1940s and early
'50s inadequate sanitary conditions at Kew resembled those found
in areas designated as urban slums such as Collingwood and Fit-
zroy. In the 1950s the Victorian Government introduced slum rec-
lamation programs to modernise the city and improve the quality
of life for people in the mainstream community. The chairman of
the Mental Hygiene Authority, Eric Cunningham Dax, demanded
similar government action for people housed in public mental
institutions.

On his first visit to Kew Cottages, Cunningham Dax was
appalled by the sanitation facilities, 'Kew Cottages is on the slope,
and there's a drain from top to bottom, the children were empty-
ing their bladders and I would have thought their bowels as well
down this drain and it just flowed down, and the stench, the smell
of the whole place was so awful.'[9] During his tour through the communal toilet blocks, he noted with disgust that excreta was not
easily flushed out through the drainage system and sewerage emp-
tied into nearby fields where cattle were feeding. When recounting

details of a subsequent fire which burnt down one of the Kew toilet blocks his humane feelings for the residents were apparent, 'it was set on fire, I don't know who did it but it was a great thing. The story was that the Matron did it!'[10] This fire and reforms at Kew in the 1950s and '60s resulted in new, improved facilities being built. However, these were still shared spaces where privacy was not provided. It would take several more decades before individual toilets were provided for the majority of Kew residents.

Up until the late 1960s, one of the major hurdles for new staff members was overcoming the confronting conditions which lay before them. Like many other newcomers, Kurt Kraushofer's first day as a ward assistant, in 1959, was a baptism of fire:

> The first day, that was a culture shock. I was working in a unit which in today's time you would say it's Dickensian … We had 36 young males (mostly in their 20s). They were dressed in a 'combination' where you put your hands in and your feet in and two press studs in the back … I was put in the little room which wasn't more than three metres by four metres. They were sitting on a bench and I was on the entrance. There was no exit, one door only with a bucket, and they were sitting the whole day there … peeing and defecating … The meal came three times a day and they were fed sitting there … Then they went in the bathroom, 36 males. We had to basically pull these bloody plunkets off them because they were caked onto their behinds and put them into the shower. There were two showers for 36 people and one bath, so you can imagine. It wasn't a pleasure for them and it was even a lesser pleasure for somebody like me. I had never experienced those things in my life and it was a shock to the system … I've never seen so much faeces in my life than what I seen over there in one day.[11]

Personal circumstances meant that Kurt could not consider leaving his job at the Cottages, however others were repulsed by the conditions and fled from Kew never to return.

Conditions in the bathrooms were also unsatisfactory. Ted Rowe was not fond of the close supervision or showering en masse. He recalled that in the, 'big shower room … eight goes in a time and they time you. They say "Righto, time to get out of the shower and dry yourself and go to your dormitory to get your clothes on."'[12]

Patrick Reed shuddered when he described showering in the 50s and 60s, 'they used to have old, real old showers ... and sometimes the water's cold, sometimes hot'.[13] Bathing regimes altered during different eras and were dependent on the timetable associated with a particular ward. Nursing sister, Irene Harvey, remembered that in the 1920s showering was often a weekly activity.[14] She was adamant that this practice did not reflect a deliberate attempt to deny residents basic hygiene standards, but was customary in the general community, 'in our world when we were children, we had a bath once [a week] ... it wasn't anything unusual'.[15] From the late 1950s many residents were taken to the bathroom to wash daily, while others, mostly residents with higher support needs, were cleaned when deemed necessary by their ward staff.

During her first months at Kew, Austra Kurzeme was amazed at the speed at which nurses bathed some residents. She was expected to perform at a similar level, 'I had to learn to bath quickly, I saw some nurses just pull the child through the water, make the hair wet, the face wet, the bottom clean, and dry and put some powder on, and then the child appeared to be bathed.'[16] Austra explained that there 'just wasn't time' to administer a thorough clean as there were so many residents who needed to be washed within strict time periods. Quality of service was hampered by understaffing and overcrowding.

Some staff were tireless in their efforts to maintain reasonable levels of hygiene within the wards. Margaret McDonald was horrified by the lack of sanitation when she worked at the Cottages in the 1940s. She devoted herself to incessantly cleaning the wards and residents. To her disdain, after only a month in one ward, she was transferred by the charge sister for cleaning too much.[17] A few staff members were indifferent towards cleanliness, allowing residents to wallow in filthy conditions. However these unhygienic conditions were potential contributors to ill-health, not only for residents, but staff as well. Despite the risk, most people felt resigned to the fact that unsanitary conditions were part and parcel of life at Kew. Until the 1960s, standards fell far short of reasonable levels of hygiene found in the general Australian community. Clearly, living in 'State care' did not accord with being adequately cared for by the State.

During the 1950s and '60s major renovations took place at the Cottages. These improvements predominantly resulted from donations received through government and public subscription from the Tipping Appeal (see Chapter 8). Dilapidated wards were renovated and new facilities were built. In addition to physical changes, the number of residents housed in each ward decreased and domestic staff were employed to assist in the wards. In recruiting domestics, institutional management hoped that nursing staff would be able to attend more directly to the care and training of residents in everyday life skills such as toileting. Maria Kraushofer discussed the reforms and staff resistance to some changes:

> The number [of residents] decreased from 80 to 60. The toilets became four and then ... they renovated the unit and so we got eight toilets ... Then a few years later, in late '60s, the unit got renovated again. The number got reduced to 40, 20 ladies went to Kingsbury. It started to be quite workable and manageable and we started to teach the girls to do certain things. Anyway we still had some [chamber] pots. Kurt was already working in the office [as a manager], and he came down and said to us: 'I want all the pots out of the units.' We said to him: 'It's not possible.' He said: 'Well I'll make sure that you will have no fun. You will only sit half an hour for your meal breaks, not 45 minutes. Unless you get rid of the pots, I'll be here all the time. Do you want me here?' Anyway I said to the girls: 'Let's get rid of the pots otherwise we don't get rid of him!' ... Once we saw that we can [sic] achieve this then we progressed slowly and slowly to other things.[18]

The eradication of the chamber pots and training residents to use toilet facilities was considered by Maria and Kurt to be a great improvement in ward living conditions. Years later, they were both frustrated and saddened when staff and policy changes resulted in a reversion of toileting and sanitary conditions. Maria stated that after she left, 'the pots got back in. After 15 years they started doing it on the floor, the carpet was ripped out, they sat on the floor with their legs open'.[19] It would appear that even with the determination of some staff to enact positive reforms these could be easily reverted through the actions of fellow staff members who failed to uphold standards of care.

Until the late 20th century, bathing and showering were mechanical, public activities where residents were literally herded through bathrooms like cattle. On his first day working as a unit staff member, in 1986, Michael Glenister was surprised by the public nature of personal care, 'You get in there at seven o'clock in the morning and there are 30 fellas who want to have a shower and they just stripped off ready for a shower, but they're wandering around, up and down the hallway, in and out of the bathroom, and in the lounge-room and yes it's just bizarre'.[20] A lack of personal space and attention persisted into the 21st century and was noted by a community visitor, 'it was reported to me by a student on placement here once that in one unit there were, I'll try and be conservative, say 28 ladies, that were all showered in 13 minutes in the morning'.[21]

The impersonal nature of showering and bathing was compounded by the physical make-up of the facilities. Steven Wears, a resident from 1962–2006, explained that he washed in a big room forthrightly declaring, 'everybody was in the shower, everybody'.[22] By the 1990s stalls were erected with doors attached for greater privacy in many units. In a focus group held in 2006, some community visitors were critical of this set-up, as the following extract demonstrates:

VISITOR the big shower rooms ... are clean in a sense, but they've deteriorated physically and there's ... this huge room and a shower in the corner and a basin and the gumboots.

VISITOR The [staff] gumboots!

VISITOR I always think, if you put me in there and gave me showers, I'd feel like a horse in a stall. It's really what it looks like.[23]

After enduring communal showers for decades, many residents welcomed the improved, private facilities. Ralph Dawson was one such resident who, when asked about the newer bathrooms, stated that he liked them because 'We had privacy ... We had walls.'[24] The introduction of private facilities features strongly in residents' stories. Even though many residents grew up in a world where activities were done collectively, they desired and valued personal time and space. Residents were often quick to remark that privacy was the greatest benefit of moving out of Kew and into community housing. Although this response could be attributed to staff influence, as this is a common benefit championed by many institutional staff in regards to community rehousing, this sentiment appeared genuine as many residents have spoken of 'bad times' when private moments did not exist.

The running of a large institution such as Kew Cottages depended upon residents being cared for and directed in groups. Communality in personal care extended into their physical appearance. Up until the 1980s, the majority of residents were dressed in items stored in collective wardrobes. These clothes were often 'government issue' or cast-offs donated from a variety of organisations including the Army and football clubs.[25] The type of clothing resembled that used at other institutions, such as orphanages and prisons. Economic factors largely determined the quality and style of attire. Nurse, Julie Carpenter, recalled that when she started at the Cottages in 1977, 'The clothing at Kew was very institutional. When I first came they were dressed in government clothing. The boys had grey shorts and anyone that might run away wore a red t-shirt so that you could see them as they dashed off down the paddock. I was quite shocked.'[26] The uniformity of residents' appearance allowed Kew Cottages to be a controlled environment where staff were easily identifiable from residents.

The use of communal clothing was not only a practical consideration, as staff policing of an individual's personal belongings was not feasible, but also reflected ways in which institutions de-personalised residents.[27] This approach ensured that essential services such as laundry were easier to deliver and that possible tensions between residents about ownership of clothing were averted.

Ted Rowe recalled that in the 1920s and '30s he wore 'just ordinary clothes like prison clothes'; a calico shirt and trousers that were 'like jeans'.[28] These were most likely moleskin trousers which were standard issue at that time. Boots were commonplace. At night time pyjamas were worn:

TED They call them pyjamas.

CORINNE What were they like?

TED Bloody awful!

CORINNE What was awful about them?

TED They were rough, you could feel them on your skin.

CORINNE They were a scratchy, rough material?

TED Yeah, scratchy. They'd got lines in them like you're out on the football field.[29]

When I asked Ted if he received new clothes regularly he replied, 'they got replaced when they had holes in them and that. They sent them out and they might be able to repair them on the machine and bring them back to you but otherwise you get a new pair. But they wouldn't wear out, they were like sheet iron.'[30] Hard-wearing clothes were essential for the institution, as it had very limited resources to purchase these items. In general, frugality outweighed comfort.

For many staff, functionality was the most important aspect for clothing residents. Ward assistant, Ted Wilson, recalled that in the 1940s and '50s the residents:

> were much easier to undress in those days. No shoes, no socks. Moleskin pants and Army coats. No underwear. Castings off from the Army. But what was worse than no shoes or socks was when they brought in the old thick socks and Army boots, when you had to lace up 110 boots with leather laces … the patients get diarrhoea in the first couple of hours and you have to undo them again.[31]

Ted Wilson was critical about the shirts and trousers supplied as both relied on buttons for fastening and attaching braces. The rough

Destruction of Clothing

Although the standard of clothing at Kew
Cottages was often poor, sometimes it was not
the fault of the institution. Some residents were
infamous for destroying or shedding clothing
when the opportunity arose. Ripping clothes,
popping buttons and discarding shoelaces
were the most common forms of destruction.
Sometimes these behaviours were the direct
result of defiance or an attempt to relieve
the monotony of institutional life. At other
times these acts were a means of expressing
frustration or communicating a problem with a
particular item of clothing. Whatever the reason,
destruction of clothing was a major problem
in some areas of Kew. In the 1970s, Dianne
Pymble worked in a unit with a group of female
teenagers. She recalled, 'When I donated my
dresses to the unit, most were ripped within a day
of them being worn.'

(Dianne Pymble, 'Written Recollections', Kew Cottages History
Project, La Trobe University, 22 September 2006.)

treatment of clothing, by both the laundry staff and many residents,
meant that buttons which came off were not often sewn on again.
Shirts were sometimes missing all of the buttons leaving residents
looking dishevelled and exposed to the elements. Many staff members
believed that clothing such as pants with an elastic waistband would
have been more suitable for residents. Unhappy with the clothing
supplied at Kew, Ted Wilson complained directly to Cunningham
Dax during one of his visits to the Cottages. He pleaded, 'Do us a
favour; no buttons, no braces and no laces!'[32]

A paucity of suitable clothing was a common gripe among staff at Kew. Staff would sometimes fight to secure the best clothing for their charges. A community visitor stated, 'Someone told me about the underwear, about everyone not having their own underwear and the staff rushing to get the best underwear for *their* person.'[33] Nurse, Margaret McDonald, claimed 'I used to fight for clothes for them with the old charge sister. She'd get very haughty and I'd get just as haughty.'[34]

In the 1930s and 1940s most Australians suffered from hard economic times and wartime rationing. From the 1950s, economic growth resulted in prosperity for many people in the mainstream community. Consumerism was burgeoning with an emphasis on fashion and recreational living. At Kew Cottages the prevalence of children and adults dressed in poor clothing, many without foot-wear, starkly contrasted with the middle-class idealism of this era. Being locked away in an institution, the residents were virtually invisible to the world at large.

By the 1970s, clothing standards were little improved. Ruth Anghie was shocked at the calico underpants that many of the older girls and women were wearing and the pyjama style trousers that were newly purchased as day-wear for some male residents. On viewing the trousers she confronted the manager in charge and suc-cessfully demanded that new pants be ordered that reflected those worn by people in the mainstream community.[35] In the 1980s, when residents and staff were eventually given the power to select and buy clothing, standards increased and individuality in appearance emerged at Kew. Former chief executive officer of Kew, Max Jack-son, remembered:

> Throughout the '80s there was a gradual move towards individual dress, where nurses would take the clients out to buy their own clothes as opposed to simply getting tracksuits out of the [Kew Cottages'] Store ... the ladies would have their hair done and makeup would be applied.[36]

Individuality of dress was a fundamental change that not only impacted on the physical appearance of residents, but encouraged

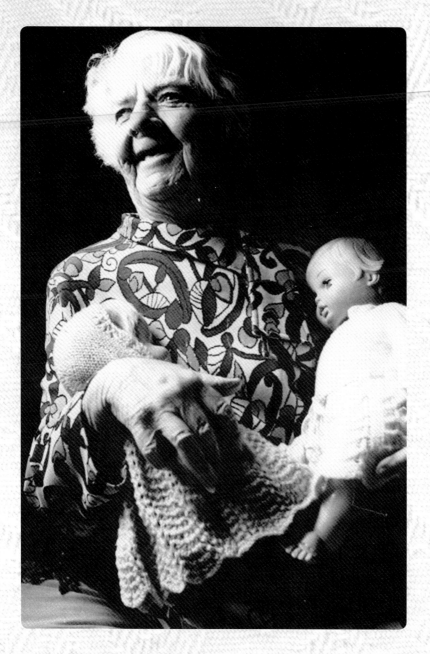

A resident dressed in her best outfit and proudly displaying her dolls, which were prized possessions, 1975. (Courtesy of Kew Residential Services, Department of Human Services, Victoria)

staff, volunteers and families to foster greater interaction between residents and members of the general community. Helen Wilson recalled, 'When they (residents) started getting paid the pension … they were able to actually go and purchase their own clothing, or staff went and did it on their behalf. They had their own clothes and they started to look nice. They were more presentable, people were more willing to go out and about with them when they looked more respectable.'[37] The responsibility of acquiring clothing for residents was taken very seriously by some staff, such as nurse Wilma Keller who often bought clothes from one of Melbourne's leading department stores. Even though residents had the potential to choose their own clothing, this right was mostly enjoyed by those who were able to easily communicate their wishes. Other residents were left to the whim of families and staff to make decisions. Consequently, the fashion styles of some residents closely resembled the clothes worn by people in control of clothing purchases.

Residents who were interviewed take pride in their appearance. On many occasions I was shown new clothing purchases at our meetings. For example David Honner was very proud of his bright white runners, while Donald Starick modelled new jumpers that he bought. Shopping for clothes and freedom of choice was important for many residents. Patrick Reed stated that he enjoyed going to Bob Stewart's Menswear, 'I used to go down to Kew Junction … the staff from the Cottages took us.'[38] A few clothing shops also sent personnel to the Cottages to cater for residents who were not assisted in shopping outside of the institution. When buses were introduced at Kew, shopping trips for residents were frequently scheduled. This gave them the opportunity to access retail outlets in the local area and larger shopping centres. Clothing options expanded significantly and greater individuality ensued.

During the early period of moving towards greater individualisation, in association with clothing changes, residents were also able to access hairdressing salons and barber shops in the community. Before this era residents relied mostly on untrained staff or securing the services of a visiting hairdresser. Maria Kraushofer recalled helping the ladies in her unit with their hair and make-up before attending social events such as dances, 'we had a hairdressing room ... which on the day of the dance, we started grooming in the morning, put the curlers in their hair'.[39] In later years a hairdressing salon was set up at Kew. Jan Sharp, a former hairdresser, worked in administration and was responsible for establishing this facility. She recalled that it was a successful venture that gave enjoyment to residents who utilised this service.[40]

Photographs taken from the 1970s appear to show individuality emerging among residents at Kew Cottages. Despite these apparent advances, in 2007 schedules continued to dominate the nature of life at the Cottages. Even though most of us have daily personal care routines and timetables, these are not usually communal in nature. Over time the number of residents being designated into groups vastly decreased, yet treatment of them as individuals, with different tastes and desires, often remained sadly lacking.

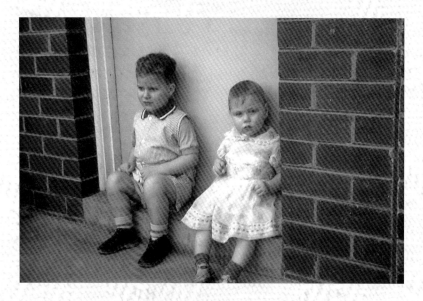

Two of Kew's young residents, circa 1965. Many residents were dressed up when their photos were to be taken. (Courtesy of Kew Cottages Historical Society)

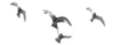

Shepherd's Pie to Stir Fry

As to the meal, there was a tin of porridge, tin of sliced bread (the nurses put butter, jam and peanut butter on), some mince, and nurses made 'sop' – cut up bread and pouring milk on top. When the bread was soaked – it was ready to eat. And then [the] charge nurse or second nurse poured from a big bottle some white stuff to the mixture – I never managed to find out what it was. Some said it was against diarrhoea, but to my knowledge there was more diarrhoea after eating sop with this stuff mixed in.

Austra Kurzeme, Kew staff, circa 1987

Up until 1993, Kew Cottages relied upon a central kitchen to produce meals. As the number of residents and staff increased throughout the decades, pressure on the kitchen also intensified. As in other areas of the Cottages, the kitchen ran on a skeleton staff and operated on a minimal budget. The provision of meals at Kew was based upon the ideal of human necessity, rather than residents' enjoyment or wellbeing. As a State-run institution, Kew Cottages often failed in its duty of care to provide residents with basic levels of quality food and service. Many residents suffered from health problems directly associated with malnutrition. In the 1960s and '70s, major food service reforms took place due to the efforts of a handful of concerned staff who demanded improvements. From the 1980s further changes resulted as institutional policy shifted. However for much of its history, Kew Cottages residents were deprived of a nutritional diet and a congenial atmosphere in which to enjoy meals.

Cooking meals at Kew revolved around meeting budgets and timetables. As finances were strictly limited, substandard food items were often bought and up until the mid-20th century were supplemented by produce obtained from the farm located at the Kew Mental Hospital. In the 1920s and '30s, Ted Rowe worked on the farm, 'We used to have … a roster. They'd [staff] come in and say "You've got to milk the cows this morning." I said "Right oh" and I went down and milked. I had three cows to milk … and [staff would shout] "Don't drink the milk!"'[1] Although used for therapeutic purposes, the farm also served a vital role in contributing to the diet of people associated with both the Mental Hospital and Cottages.

At different times in Kew's history staff were accused of stealing from the institution's kitchen supplies. In his autobiography, Reginald Ellery, a medical officer at Kew from 1923–26, wrote that among staff 'Pilfering was not uncommon. Some of the food delivered for the patients found its way to the attendants' homes.'[2] Similarly, Ruth Anghie reported that this type of activity occurred in the 1970s, 'There was a lot of theft, things were taken straight from the kitchen.'[3] Allegations of theft were rarely reported to senior management or investigated. One exception was in the 1990s, when Jan Sharp was appointed to investigate the catering accounts. After three weeks of investigation, she concluded that no misappropriation had occurred.[4]

Generally, kitchen staff were not required to have professional cooking or catering skills. Staffing levels were low requiring the assistance of resident labour. Ted Wilson recalled that in the 1940s two cooks were supported by eight to 10 residents.[5] The menus were

basic fare such as porridge and shepherd's pie that could be produced efficiently en masse. A lack of concern over food standards
was not only evidenced in the management's willingness to recruit
untrained kitchen staff, but in its secondment of nursing and ward
staff to work in this area. In the 1950s, Sylvia Babic was ordered
by the matron in her ward to replace a cook who was going on
leave. She was required to cater for two wards of people who were
on special diets. Sylvia admitted that her own cooking skills were
questionable at the best of times, but felt compelled to take on her
new role. After being handed a menu, she was expected to prepare
meals without assistance from the other two 'elderly cooks'. Sylvia
wrote, 'some days the porridge would be like soup, whilst on others
it would be so you could almost jump on it … Finally my time in
the kitchen came to an end and I was glad, and more than likely so
were the wards.'[6] Residents had very few avenues for making their
complaints heard when served substandard food. One of the most
common forms of protest was refusing to eat. By rejecting the food,
residents exposed themselves to possible negative repercussions
including hunger or punishment by staff for causing trouble. With
so many mouths to feed within a set time period, many staff did not
tolerate such rebelliousness.

At mealtimes staff supervision was ever-present and vigilant.
Ted Rowe noted, 'Some of them wouldn't eat it. They used to shove
it over, "Here, here, you can have this". [If you were caught, the staff
would shout –] "What are you doing there?" God, they've got eyes
like a hawk, some of them. "Oh he's just showing me what his food's
like".'[7] The chairman of the Mental Hygiene Authority, Eric Cunningham Dax, was aware of the oppressive and tense atmosphere
for residents in the dining hall, 'when you went in at mealtimes
they were sitting at the tables, on benches usually, as you went past
they put their hands over their ears because if they weren't eating
their food they got a clip over the ear'.[8] Clare Turner confirmed that
rough treatment prevailed in the 1960s. Clare recalled that on more
than one occasion when she refused to eat her porridge the staff
'make me, slapped me across, across, the face'.[9] The domineering

attitude of some staff, in combination with the serving of inferior food, made mealtimes a time of endurance, rather than a pleasure, for many residents.

The majority of Kew residents ate in large groups assembled in a central dining area or in the wards. Ted Rowe ate in the central dining hall, where the food 'Wasn't bad. Could have had better, but they don't give you much.'[10] At times the small serves were a blessing, particularly in regards to the morning porridge, commonly known as 'the glue'. Ted recalled that breakfast was, 'always porridge ... We always used to say "Oh you got this glue out again!"'[11] Up until the 1970s, lunch was the main meal of the day. Meat, mostly mince, and vegetables were the staple food items accompa-

Black Tablecloth

Not only was the standard of food considered to be poor at Kew Cottages, the levels of basic hygiene in food preparation and service were also questionable. When the chairman of the Mental Hygiene Authority, Dr Eric Cunningham Dax, visited Kew in 1952, he was horrified by the conditions he found:

I'd been to numerous hospitals in England and in other countries, but I'd never seen anything like Kew Cottages ... I remember going to one ward and there was the table there and I thought it had a black tablecloth on it, but this is true, I'm not exaggerating, they were flies. I think it was the remains of some of the dinner that they'd had which were over the table, and all these flies had settled down, and it was black, all over the top, you can't believe it.

(Interview with Dr Eric Cunningham Dax, 9 January 2006)

nied by dessert. In the evening, at 5 pm, refreshments such as soup and toast were provided, sometimes with the option of something sweet, such as fruit, when available. Morning and afternoon tea, were not introduced until the end of the 20th century. Up until the 1980s, if residents were hungry outside designated mealtimes additional food was usually not on offer. Ted Rowe stipulated, 'No, no, they won't give you any. "You had your meal", they say, "You didn't eat, well that's your fault!"'[12]

For decades the staff at Kew also ate meals that were prepared by the central kitchen. Meals were often included as a staff benefit or for a nominal fee. Nurse, Irene Harvey, referred to the meals as 'tolerable … as meals cooked in large numbers are … we wouldn't like them much now!'[13] Up until the 1960s male and female staff ate separately. Irene noted, 'I do remember distinctly in the old nurses' mess room, up there on the hill, there was the males' mess room and the females' mess room.'[14] It would appear that the gender segregation that existed among residents in the institution was also imposed upon staff facilities. The staff dining area was relocated as the institution evolved and eating arrangements changed as the gender barriers broke down. On a few occasions residents, such as Patrick Reed, also had the privilege of eating among staff. Patrick loved his Friday lunches, 'I'd go up to the kitchen … [where] all the staff used to go … I used to go up and get fish and chips every Friday.'[15] At that time Patrick was working in the Cottages' Stores area and was able to enjoy privileges associated with his status as a worker.

A minority of staff who were sympathetic towards the plight of residents brought in additional food supplies. In the 1940s, school teacher, Evelyn Richards, used food as an incentive for her students to behave. On occasion she also distributed food to residents housed in nearby wards. According to Evelyn, her mother regularly baked special treats for the residents such as cakes, biscuits and scones. If these were unavailable then Evelyn brought in bread and butter.[16] The recipients of such kindness were in the minority and those most directly associated with a particular staff member, others were not so lucky. From the 1960s, with residents being given access to money through pensions and small wages, some frequented the onsite kiosk to purchase special indulgences unavailable in the wards. When I asked Nick Konstantaras if he bought coffee at the kiosk, he replied 'sometimes ... but Coke's better'.[17] Wendy Pennycuick told me that she would buy 'lollies ... and drinks'.[18] Luxury food items were enjoyed by residents who were able to purchase these goods or who were privy to the kindness of others. Institutional food was mostly basic fare.

The blatant disregard for residents' enjoyment of food at Kew was highlighted in the strange food combinations and work practices of some staff. Kurt Kraushofer revealed:

> One of my worst experiences, it was late '50s, early '60s, when food came from a central kitchen. It was mainly mince, mince and teacake, and the mince was boiling hot, so what do you do? You chuck the milk in it to cool it off [and] then it's too thin. What do you do then? You put the teacake in it. That's how I was told to do it and when you're brand new you can't speak out, you do it, and the whole lot was put on a plate and we fed them. Those type of things disappeared over a while but that's how tough it was for clients.[19]

Andrew Ledwidge confirmed Kurt's claim stating that he was often served 'sloppy kitchen food'.[20]

Even in the 21st century, a few insensitive staff continued to mix food items in a manner that would be considered peculiar, even unacceptable, in mainstream society. In 2006, community visitors witnessed this unusual behaviour in a Kew unit and publicly brought it to the attention of management:

VISITOR All of the ladies were having their brunch, so we stood at the door not to intrude on their meals ... they were having weak milky tea, which of course 'everyone likes', in the jug, nothing individual ... it was brunch, sausages, baked beans and omelette, but all mashed up together into a mess ... and they got half way through their weak milky tea and the carer went to the fridge, got out a great big bottle of prune juice and just went around and sloshed the prune juice into everyone's tea.

VISITOR It's a cocktail, it's popular! [said mockingly]

VISITOR I nearly gagged, I had to walk away, that's about the most disgusting thing I've ever seen. I'm not kidding!

VISITOR 'You've got to be regular.' [indicating staff attitude]

VISITOR Yesterday at the quarterly meeting, I brought a couple of little bottles of prune juice and invited the management if they'd like to put some in their tea.

VISITOR It was brilliant.

CORINNE Did anyone take it up?

VISITOR No, but the picture was beautiful.[21]

The communal plastic jug of tea and doling out of prune juice were symbolic of the ways in which residents' personal preferences or tastes were often disregarded at Kew Cottages. Institutional life revolved around the administration of groups, often at the expense of the individual.

From its early history malnourishment was a constant concern at Kew, for without a proper diet many residents suffered health problems. In 1959, paediatrician, David Pitt, discovered widespread dental sepsis, nutritional anaemia, worm infestations and a few cases of scurvy.[22] In response to the endemic health issues created by poor food service, a group of senior staff including David, secretary Des Nugent, caterer Harold Reid and dentist George Harris, formed a committee to upgrade the residents' diet. David argued that, 'Improving the diet was important. A lot of the children had anaemia from iron deficiency … [and] were infested with intestinal worms … the worms were due to an excessive carbohydrate diet.'[23] The committee decided to increase protein meals from two to three a day, provide more fruit and administer vitamin supplements to vulnerable residents.[24] David claimed that by implementing these changes, dental and general health slowly improved and worm infestations vanished. These alterations were significant in

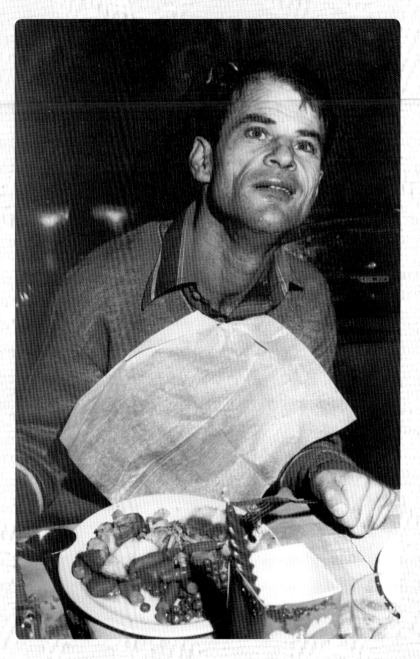

A resident eating his meal in Unit 11, 1977. (Courtesy of Kew Residential Services, Department of Human Services, Victoria)

overcoming some of the health problems present at the institution, but others persisted.

In the 1970s, Ruth Anghie was suspicious about the standard of food being given to residents, particularly the mince meat:

> If you looked at the menu, because the menus used to be sent out, you would have thought you were in a four-star or five-star hotel, all fancy names, but it was the same sort of thing; mince disguised in various ways. The mince was causing a lot of diarrhoea. In one unit there were twin boys. I ended up having to write on their histories that they were *never* to be given mince because they were getting diarrhoea as a result of the mince.[25]

Unable to 'officially' have the food tested, Ruth conspired with technicians at the local laboratory to test samples of food that she mislabelled 'faeces'. According to Ruth, these diagnostic tests revealed the mince to be riddled with a type of bacteria that was associated with repeated and inadequate reheating. She did not support the directive which required staff to return all uneaten food to the kitchen in order for it to be recycled, instead she instructed staff in her units to throw uneaten or inadequately prepared food into the 'pig-bin'.

Ruth was not averse to storming up to the superintendent's office with a plate of food demanding that something be done to improve standards. On one occasion she asked Dr Gary McBrearty, '"Could you eat this? Would you give it to your children? If the answer is 'no', then it's not good enough for the residents here!"'[26] Ruth also considered that mealtimes were too early and that the main meal should be given in the evening. After consulting with unit staff, she successfully put her case forward to senior management to alter these arrangements. The health status of some residents improved through these changes. Ruth explained, 'by giving the meals later, medications were also given later as they were usually given with meals. This reduced the early morning seizures that many of the residents [experienced] who suffered with epilepsy'.[27]

Ruth was motivated to seek food service reforms after observing first-hand the culinary skills of Kew kitchen staff:

I think it was in my second year there, there was an interstate conference on retardation and psychiatry, and people came from all over for two days. We had lunch provided, and when I went for that lunch, I couldn't believe my eyes! It was such a spread of beautiful food and produced from Kew kitchen. You name it; every meat was there, suckling pig with the apple in the mouth and salads. I thought: 'I wonder what the kids are getting?' I knew then, you have cooks who can cook, so why isn't the food better? It was then that I started fighting.[28]

It would appear that during this period kitchen staff were highly skilled. However catering to the needs of over 900 residents three times a day was vastly different from providing lunch for a smaller conference group. The act of efficiently and regularly producing hundreds of meals was often the goal of kitchen staff, rather than providing high quality food. This attitude reflected the economic stringency that governed the administration of many State facilities.

Nurse, Julie Carpenter, considered that even in the late 1970s the diet and provision of food at Kew was substandard. She believed that drastic improvements in nutrition and feeding practices were desperately needed. Julie claimed that 'Mealtimes used to be quite traumatic, for a lot of them, they were inadequately fed ... Some food was inedible. You'd get meat that was so tough you couldn't cut it.'[29] When Max Jackson worked at the Cottages in the late 1970s and '80s, he was critical of the state of the food service:

One of the big problems with Kew is its huge grounds, and institutions tend to be dictated by the routine of staff, the industrial requirements and rosters. Nurses worked a 12-hour shift so they would come on at seven o'clock in the morning and there'd be a changeover at around seven or 7.30 at night. It meant that things like your meals, evening meal for example would be served probably about five o'clock. The reason for that would be so that the clients could be bathed and put into their 'jammies', by about half past five. It was one of the real negatives of an institution, when you saw adults roaming around the grounds or sitting outside the units rocking or inside rocking, in their pyjamas at about half past five, quarter to six at night. But that was dictated by the food services.[30]

Max recognised that the structure and administration of the

institution were key problems in providing reasonable levels of food service:

> There was a central kitchen plating eight or nine hundred meals, the units didn't have cooking facilities as such, and so the meals would be transported around by a little tractor type arrangement with a carriage behind with the meals sitting in the carriage in hot-boxes. Of course many of the roads and footpaths around Kew weren't all that smooth and so by the time the food got to the units the custard would probably be mixed with the gravy and it was pretty atrocious.[31]

When he accepted the position of CEO at Kew in 1984, Max worked alongside other senior managers to overhaul this area. Not only was transportation of food an issue, so too the quality of produce being bought. As with most institutions, purchasing cheap cuts of meat and other produce was standard practice. Max said that under his leadership Kew took 'a more stringent approach to meal preparation and rather than

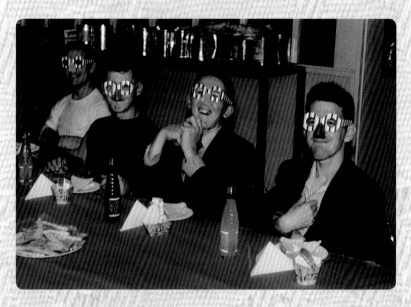

Residents sometimes received specialty
food items to celebrate occasions such
as birthdays, Easter and Christmas.
Kew Cottages, 1961. (Courtesy of Kew
Cottages Historical Society)

the caterer buying the cheapest cuts of meat with lots of fat on it, we started to look at better cuts of meat, and fruit in the units and cooking breakfasts in the units. It was all a very gradual process.[32]

In 1991, a public scandal erupted when the president of the Kew Cottages Parents' Association, Geoff Welchman, revealed that residents were going hungry because of funding cuts, 'At Kew Cottages they are spending $3.04 on each client on a daily basis … I have been involved in servicing hostels for 12 years and the average is $5.50.'[33] Geoff argued that many residents were losing weight, including his own son, as a result of the decrease in quality and quantity of food. Some residents were purchasing food in order to satisfy hunger. The Minister of Community Services, Kay Setches, responded swiftly to Geoff's allegations and additional funding and services were allocated to this area of care. By 1995, conditions had not improved greatly. In a letter to the editor of *The Age* newspaper, parent, Rosalie Trower, was scathing of the Victorian Government claiming that the 'Daily food allowance at Kew Cottages is considerably less than daily food allowance for prisoners.'[34] It would appear that residents were continually penalised by institutional living.

Although a dietitian was employed at Kew, it was primarily the responsibility of the central kitchen and unit staff to prepare nutritious and inviting meals for residents. Quality assurance was often at the discretion of these staff members, although unannounced inspections could take place by senior staff and others such as the community visitors. In 1993, changes in institutional practice resulted in some food preparation being carried out within units for smaller numbers of residents. Michael Glenister worked in a unit when this devolution occurred:

> There was a dietitian who oversaw the whole process and made sure that … if there were any special [dietary] requirements that you would oversee that side of things, but other than that … it was completely open to the staff to shop and to cook … all of a sudden these residents who have had relatively bland food prepared en masse were being cooked for by the latest influx of migrants who

were working at Kew, that happened to be Filipino. So they were all having these curries and noodle dishes ... but there wasn't a lot of scope for the residents there to have a lot of input into what they were eating either, which is sad too, because that's one of the things people enjoy doing is to choose food that they like.[35]

Changes in food service improved the variety of food available, but residents were still reliant upon dedicated staff to ensure that their meals were well-conceived, prepared and delivered. As Michael indicated, staff predominantly catered for groups according to their own cooking styles and abilities. Although the diet had changed largely from shepherd's pie to stir fry, this was not because of resident demands, but rather staff preferences and a shift in institutional operation.

On 18 November 2005, the central kitchen permanently closed. During its 118-year history, understaffing and inadequate resources meant that food quality was often inferior to that available in mainstream Australian society. Although improvements in food service were made from the 1960s, residents were still fed according to institutional guidelines. Despite efforts to create more active engagement in food preparation and delivery through unit-based cooking, staff mostly determined the menus with little or no consultation with residents. The continued presence of the communal plastic tea jug in 2007 poignantly illustrates that residents continue to be treated as a collective group. The assumption that all residents have the same tastes and desires reveals some of the ways that institutionalisation at Kew is still alive and well in the 21st century.

CHAPTER 6

At the Heart of Kew's History

Histories that document life inside State institutions such as Kew Cottages, rarely foreground the experience of residents. The following collection of vignettes has been written to enhance residents' stories of institutional living at Kew. Each resident who was interviewed for this oral history, and who did not require a pseudonym, is represented in an individual cameo. These accounts reflect the journey of each resident and issues that they considered to be important during their time at Kew. The central location of the vignettes within this book signifies their pivotal place at the heart of Kew Cottages' history.

Edward (Ted) Rowe[1]

In 1921, Ted Rowe was abandoned in a park and was sent to live in a government institution for neglected children known as 'The Depot'. In 1925, at the age of four, Ted was transferred to Kew Cottages. Various reasons were recorded for his transfer, including 'he laughs merrily at everything and at nothing'.

When Ted arrived at Kew over 400 people were living at the institution. He recalled that male and female residents were forbidden to fraternise outside the gaze of institutional staff, '[they] put a

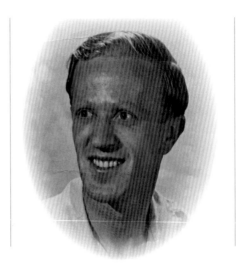

Ted Rowe, circa 1950. (Courtesy of
Edward Rowe, private collection)

division in between us, the girls on one side of the fence and us ...
on the other side'. Ted lived in a dormitory which housed up to 40
boys. Having lived in institutions virtually from birth, this lifestyle
was not a culture shock.

Ted was fortunate in being part of an elite group of residents at
the Cottages who received formal education and vocational training. He attended school and was proud of being the 'teacher's pet'.
Ted flourished at Kew and soon learned to read and write. As a
'resident worker', Ted was employed in menial jobs around the
institution.

Ted enjoyed his time at the Cottages, making the most of opportunities. His only major complaint was that there was, 'not much
good food'. One of worst culinary offenders was the morning porridge, 'We called it "the glue".' Although Ted was content at Kew, he
was determined to 'get out' as soon as possible. He said to the Kew
staff, 'I want to work, to go out and work.'

At the age of 14, Ted's development qualified him for a transfer
to Travancore Special School. In 1939, he was excited at the news
that he had a job as a farm labourer in Stawell. Ted recalled being

disappointed with his employer, 'He drive me mad, he was a slave driver.'

In 1941, Ted enlisted to fight in World War II. He was plunged into a hellish world as he was stationed in Darwin during the Japanese bombings. He said that it was 'Terrible. Damned terrible ... Every night you'd get ready to go to bed, and the siren's going, you can't sleep after that, and they're dropping bombs all the time.'

After the war, Ted married and over the years he gained employment in a pub, shoe factory and finally as a janitor at Ballarat East High School, where he worked for 25 years. Kew Cottages had equipped him with the requisite skills to survive in mainstream Australian society.

Lois Philmore[2]

Lois Philmore was first admitted to Kew Cottages in 1941 at the age of five. She was transferred from St Anthony's Home, an orphanage in Kew. A year later she was sent to live at Janefield, a training centre for people with intellectual disability located in Bundoora, but was readmitted to the Cottages in 1964.

Lois belonged to a privileged group of residents who were commonly referred to as the 'working girls'. This group were used mostly as unpaid labour to support the running of the Cottages. Lois performed cleaning duties in her ward, 'I used to clean the windows ... [and] I take me own sheets off [the bed].'

Lois recalled that when she was paid she had to house her money carefully as theft was a major problem. 'I did have my money, yes, in the dormitory ... but [Caroline Porter] ... she stole me money ... I told Miss Lucas ... she got into trouble.' The money was duly returned and Caroline reprimanded for her actions.

Like many of the 'resident workers' Lois took pride in her appearance. She preferred to wash her own clothes by hand than risk having them ruined or disappear in Kew's laundering system, 'I washed by hand, I did them by myself ... I'd rather do it on me own, and I know that it's done.'

A job that gave Lois great pleasure was working in the Wills Street home of psychiatrist Wilfrid Brady. 'I worked hard there.' Lois was beloved by the Brady household and when they moved away from the institution Lois continued to work as their house-keeper.

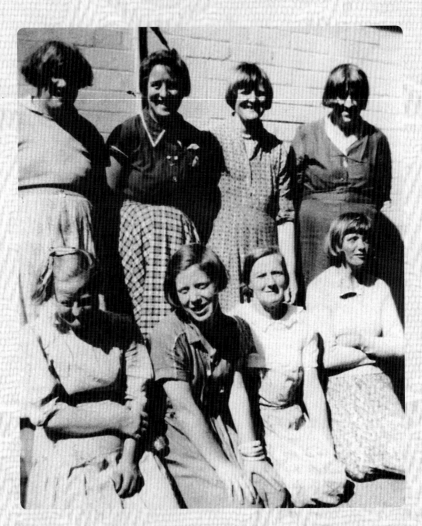

Lois Philmore (pictured in the back row second from the right) with fellow working residents at Kew Cottages, 1960s. (Courtesy of Kew Cottages Historical Society)

In 2007, Wilfrid's son, Philip, maintained a close friendship with Lois. He is proud of his long-term friendship with her, 'I'm happy to say ... that we're still really good friends and that I see her regularly ... that's a link from the past which 50 years can't erase.'

Even though Lois received special privileges, she was generally unhappy at Kew. She did not like the regimentation that governed everyday life, 'we'd got to be indoors at a certain time'. Lois was content to leave the institution, 'I wanted to move on because I'd been there for a long time.' In 1971, Lois was relocated to Moorakyne Hostel, then other shared and independent living accommodations. She supported herself through a government pension and working at VATMI (a non-profit company employing people with disabilities) in Burwood. 'I used to do the cleaning ... [then] I put the chockies [chocolates] and lollies in the bags.' Lois recognised that the life skills that she learned at Kew were valuable in supporting her independent lifestyle in later years.

Patrick Reed[3]

In 1939, Patrick Reed was born in rural Victoria. When he was two weeks old, he was placed in St Joseph's Foundling Hospital in Melbourne. Patrick spent his childhood being shunted around four different orphanages. On 9 April 1956, Patrick was admitted to Kew Cottages. He was 17 years of age.

Patrick was assigned to 'Little Pell': 'We were all in a kind of a hut, and they had a big yard around it, and you had to stay in there all day ... [It was] real cold, and no heating.' He remarked that the residents of Kew were very different from those he mixed with at the orphanages, 'they were a bit strange'.

Patrick was given 'resident worker' status. 'I started to work in the Store of Kew Cottages and then I learned to work over in the Workshop, fixing little cars.' Patrick enjoyed delivering goods from the Store around the Cottages and to the nearby Mental Hospital, 'I used to put them on the back of the train and take them around.'

Patrick said that while living at Kew he longed for open spaces,

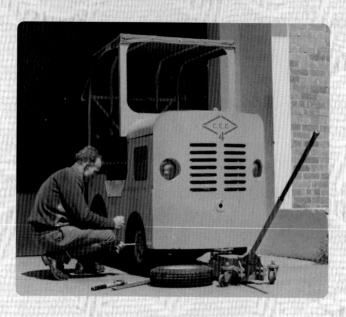

Patrick Reed changing the wheel of
a vehicle used for deliveries at Kew
Cottages, circa 1970. (Courtesy of
Patrick Reed, private collection)

'when I was working in the Store a friend said they had a bike and
they asked me did I want it and I said "yes" ... Oh I go all over the
place! ... They never find me when I was at Kew.' In later years
these journeys were made far easier after Patrick obtained his driver's licence and was given an old Ford Zephyr by the parent of a
fellow resident.

There were also times of anger and despair for Patrick while
living at Kew. He was unhappy about the rough treatment meted
out, 'I didn't like the staff ... Because they was too rough.' He also
admitted that he sometimes lashed out, particularly when staff
confiscated treasured personal belongings, 'when I was small, when
they took things off me ... I used to have a good temper, throw
things around, break windows.'

In 1981, Patrick was discharged from Kew. Since then, he has
lived in hostels and independent accommodation. He has held jobs
in places such as Jagers Carpets and Rojo Panel Beaters.

Patrick volunteered to be interviewed for this history after seeing an article about the project in his local paper. The value that Patrick places upon the history and residents' perspectives was symbolised in his donation of a CD player to the research team. Patrick stated that his donation was to allow people who did not own a player to listen to the digital history recordings. His insightful gift contributed to the decision to produce a collection of digital histories to accompany this book.

David Honner[4]

David Honner was born in New South Wales. As a young child he was sent to live in an institution at Pleasant Creek in Stawell, Victoria. In 1958, at age 14, he was transferred to Kew Cottages where he lived for 50 years.

David recalled that in his dormitory at Kew, it was 'all men all together ... [and] too noisy!' He tried to escape the chaos by going outside, 'I'd walk around, and go for a walk ... on a walker.'

David enjoyed working for many years in the Workshop, 'I made pegs *and* mops. I got paid. I bought batteries for the radio [and] I bought ice-creams and icy-poles.' He also participated in music and art programs where his creativity came to the fore.

Special occasions have been keenly celebrated by David. He has fond memories of his sister visiting and taking him out for his 60th birthday. David proudly displays a photograph taken of the two of them with his birthday cake, sparklers and candles alight.

As David grew older, he experienced balance issues that resulted in him being confined to a wheelchair, 'I'm in the wheelchair because if I use the walker now, what's going to happen? Bang! And on the ground.' He was injured on many occasions as a result of falls and received medical treatment for bone fractures and head injuries.

Sadly, David's sister passed away in 2007, he said, 'my sister's in heaven now'. He misses her as she was one of few people who came to visit. David loves company and encourages guests to spend some time with him in his unit, 'I don't mind if you stay all day.' During

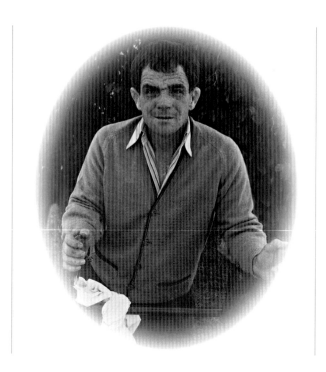

David Honner with his walker at Kew Cottages, circa 1978. (Courtesy of Kew Residential Services, Department of Human Services, Victoria)

one of our interviews he looked at me earnestly and asked, 'when I move out, are you coming to visit me or what?'

David has been saddened by Kew's demise, 'I'm not happy about it closing ... oh well ... they're closing, and what can you do?' He longs for his friends who have been relocated, 'I miss them a lot.'

David was well prepared for relocating into an onsite community residential unit with friends whom he had known for decades. He was pleased that his long time companion, Helen Wilson, was to be his house manager as they share a special bond and mutual respect for each other, 'I'm getting my own new house with Helen Wilson ... I knew Helen Wilson when I was a little baby boy ... she's been with me a long time.'

Raymond Bouker[5]

Raymond Bouker is a direct descendant of convicts Olivia Gascoigne and Nathaniel Lucas, original members of the First Fleet who were sent to colonise Norfolk Island in 1788. His family is very proud of this heritage and it is one of the first entries in Raymond's 'All About Me' book. The custodial nature of life inside Kew was rather ironic given Raymond's family history.

Born on 24 June 1954, Raymond resided at home with his parents and four siblings before being sent to live at Kew Cottages. Raymond was admitted to Ward 33 two days before he celebrated his fifth birthday, 'When I was little … Sister Zeps was there … she looked after me.' Raymond said that he did not like living at Kew as a child. When I asked why he simply stated that is was 'No good.'

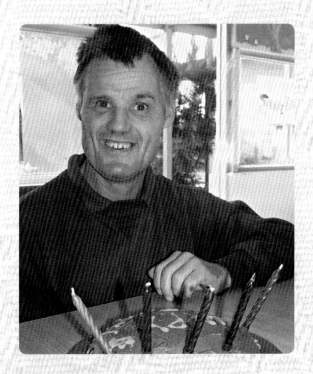

Raymond Bouker celebrating his
birthday, circa 2005. (Courtesy of
Raymond Bouker, private collection)

Raymond lived with other young boys and enjoyed attending Special School. Mathematics was one of his favourite lessons, 'I just do the sums'. Raymond still enjoys 'sums' and carries around cards with sequential numbers written on each one. He was very proud of the fact that he had been the milk monitor for his class. 'I used to go up to the kitchen, bring ... cartons of milk ... all by myself.' Raymond also helped ward staff to complete daily duties such as making up the beds 'I put the quilts down ... on the bed.'

Raymond progressed from dormitory to semi-independent and independent living accommodations. 'When I was little, 33 ... I was in Unit 1 ... I live in the hostel ... I used to be in, 26/27, for a long time ... then O'Shea.' Raymond was also sent to live outside Kew in Moorakyne Hostel for a three-month trial and was discharged to a community residential unit in 1986. Nearly three and a half years later, he was re-admitted to the Cottages after experiencing difficulties living in community housing.

With the imminent closure of Kew, Raymond was once again assigned a place in a community residential unit in 2006. This time he moved with a close-knit group of friends with whom he had lived for several years. He remarked that on driving away from Kew some of them yelled out, 'Bye-Bye Charlie!'

Although the transition into community living went smoothly, Raymond struggles to break with the regimentation that had previously dominated his life. Staff in the residential unit are actively supporting him to set aside routine and vary his activities. It would appear that his carers are making great headway as Raymond now says, 'I like it here better.'

Wendy Pennycuick[6]

The first time I interviewed Wendy Pennycuick was in a special accommodation block at Kew known as House Hostel. While we were recording, Wendy's housemates returned from their day programs. As they walked through the door they all greeted Wendy, Shirley even came over and gave her hug.

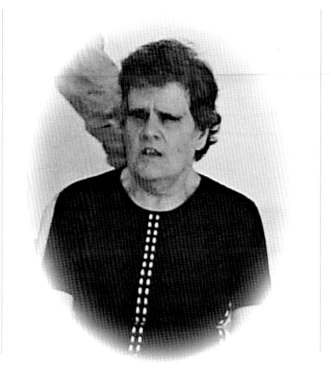

Wendy Pennycuick, circa 2000.
(Courtesy of Kew Residential Services,
Department of Human Services,
Victoria)

WENDY Here's Shirley now, Corinne.

SHIRLEY Do you want me to rub your back? (To Wendy)

WENDY Yes. She rubs my back.

CORINNE Does she rub your back, does she? And does she look after you?

SHIRLEY Yes, I do yes ... Wendy like me, Wendy like me ... she's always 'baby' to me ... I look after baby.

Wendy's face lit up as we all exchanged greetings and tales of what we'd been up to that day. It was a heart-warming scene.

Wendy was born prematurely and weighed a mere two pounds and three ounces. Oxygen deprivation associated with her prematurity resulted in blindness and intellectual disability. From the age of two, Wendy lived at the Royal Victorian Institute for the Blind (RVIB). In 1962, at eight years of age, she was transferred to Kew Cottages.

At RVIB, Wendy became friendly with a girl of similar age, Robyn Phillips. Both girls moved on to Kew and their bond of friendship has continued for almost 50 years. 'I've known Robyn for *years* … [from] a little girl … Robyn Phillips is my friend.'

Wendy received mobility training and was taught to use a cane. This aided her to navigate around Kew's grounds. On many occasions she was also guided by a companion, 'it's terrible when you can't see … Different people … help me out … it's good'.

On a winter's night in 1999, Wendy and Robyn went missing after attending an onsite advocacy meeting. 'We got lost … [we took] a wrong turn.' A search was mounted and the following morning the women were found huddled together on a local golf course. The official story is that the women wandered off, but Wendy claimed that the staff, 'sort of forgot to pick us up'. This was a frightening experience for both women.

In 2007, Wendy anxiously waited to relocate into a community residential unit that would be built onsite as part of the new housing estate. She looked forward to moving into her home with Robyn and Shirley. Wendy was aware of the delays in the redevelopment process and declared that she had to 'be patient' as these things 'take a while'.

Steven. Wears[7]

Steven Wears was admitted to the Cottages in 1962 when he was seven years old. Before this time, he had lived at home with his family. Steven explained that he stayed in contact with his family, particularly his mother, 'Tomorrow night she's going to ring [me].'

Most of his childhood was spent in the 'Schoolboys Ward' where he was assigned to the 'small boys' end. It was here that he became friendly with most of the men that he lives with today.

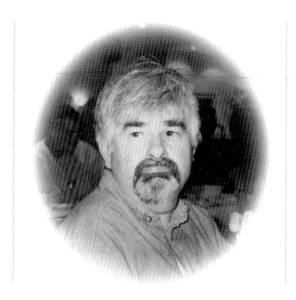

Steven Wears, circa 2002. (Courtesy of
Steven Wears, private collection)

Steven was happy when he was moved into the O'Shea building.
However, he was annoyed by the lack of cleanliness, 'Oh they never
cleaned up the place ... no-one cleans it ... I cleaned me own toilet,
and I cleaned the sink.' Steven was also proud of his role in O'Shea
as the person designated to wash clothes in the unit. 'I do everybody's washing ... every night ... straight in the washing machine
... [then] in the dryer.'

Steven was a keen sportsman who always looked forward to swimming sessions in the Sport and Recreation Centre. 'I do it myself,
went swimming. I went with Jan Sharp, but I don't do it now.' Steven
also remembered that it was sometimes difficult getting in and out
of the pool, 'There was a hoist ... It's very hard to get in.' Steven also
played soccer, 'a long time ago I played soccer ... it's not hard at all'.
Clearly, being confined to a wheelchair was not an impediment.

As he sat in the Art Room at VATMI in 2007, Steven carefully
chose different coloured markers to produce greeting cards for
public sale. He enjoyed working as an artist 'we go to work ... we do

cards ... and [wrapping] papers'. Steven had worked as an artist for many years after being taught at Kew Cottages. His paintings have been publicly exhibited and have fetched hundreds, and sometimes thousands, of dollars. 'I do the white canvas ... I do circles ... I do squares ... we draw them.' One of the images that Steven prefers to draw and paint is a tree laden with vibrant colours.

The first interview that Steven recorded for this history was three days before his relocation from Kew into a community residential unit. By this time he had lived at the Cottages for 44 years. He was excited about the move and proudly showed a picture of his new home, 'that's the house I'm going in there ... Tuesday we're going'. He said that he was 'happy' to move from Kew as his housemates were long-time friends with whom he had lived for decades.

Patricia (Patty) Rodgers[8]

Patty Rodgers was born in 1957. Patty first went to Kew when her mother was hospitalised after giving birth to a baby boy, Paul. Patty's mother was unaware that she had been sent to Kew and was furious upon her return home. She immediately organised for Patty's discharge, but within a matter of weeks Patty was re-admitted due to home pressures. She had just turned seven-years-old.

Every week, Patty's mother caught two trains and a tram on her long journey to Kew. Patty's sister, Margaret recalled the emotional devastation of visiting her sister at the Cottages, 'just going to see Patty used to be terrible because she'd scream when we left, this went on for years and years'. Patty agreed with her sister stating, 'that's right!'

For most of her time at Kew, Patty lived in shared accommodation. She helped fellow residents with daily care. She stated, 'I'd get Wendy out early in the morning ... I'd get her dressed ... and Robyn.' She made the women breakfast and also escorted them to social events such as the disco.

Living in an institution where activities tended to be collective, residents often had no choice about whether they wanted to par-

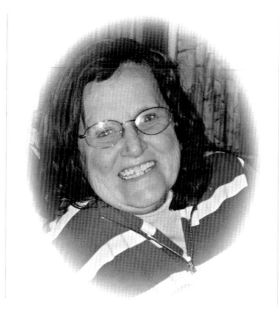

Patty Rodgers, circa 2007. (Courtesy of
Patricia Rodgers, private collection)

ticipate. Patty explained that sometimes she was forced to attend
onsite dances, 'I don't wanted to, I have to ... I don't like it.' She
said that she loved music and dancing with her friend Sally and
boyfriend Colin, but on occasion she would have preferred to stay
in the unit because it was 'too noisy'.

Patty had many friends at Kew. She enjoyed the company of
others and was happy to talk about her relationship with her current boyfriend, Colin. 'We've been girlfriends and boyfriends for
a long time ... I would take him for a walk.' Patty and Colin frequented the onsite kiosk where they met up with other friends who
lived at Kew. This was also a social place where Patty and her family
spent time.

In 1999, Patty was relocated into a community residential unit.
When I asked her what she thought about Kew Cottages and leaving she replied, 'I don't like it ... I just I hate it ... I'm happy to get
out of Kew.' Patty has been able to continue her partnership with

Colin as they now live together, 'I have my own room at the house … he comes to *me*.' Although Patty cannot move freely around her neighbourhood, as she had once done at Kew, she prefers to live in the community.

Ralph Dawson[9]

Ralph Dawson was born in South Australia in 1956. The first six weeks of his life were spent in a babies' home before he was fostered, and eventually adopted. For nine years Ralph lived on a country farm with his adoptive family. For a range of reasons, including inadequate access to special education, his parents decided to send Ralph to Kew. On 30 June 1965, he was admitted to the Cottages.

Ralph recalled that when he lived in the dormitories at Kew it was, 'Not that good … too much noise … too much boring'. Even when he had his own room in O'Shea Ralph was unhappy, 'No good … It was too small … I always fall out of the bed.'

Ralph attended school, therapy programs and the Workshop. A talented artist, he has enjoyed producing ceramic ware and art works that have fetched thousands of dollars. 'I used to work with all the art staff in Perkins.' His creativity and flamboyance are reflected in his bright and detailed paintings, especially his fish and stickmen. 'I made a fish cup … I picked the fish cup and draw on it … it was an easy one to do.'

It was not unusual to see Ralph wandering around the institutional grounds and its environs. He often walked to Kew Junction where he would buy cigarettes and sometimes beer with his wages. He recalled one particular day when, 'I had some coins in my pocket, I said: "Whacko! Let's go for a stroll, we'll going to the bottle shop." I was so lucky, I bought four, stubbies or cans.' Ralph sat outside near the bottle shop imbibing his beer. He continued his story, 'there was one man there, happy man sitting next to me, I said to him, "Here, you come sit next to me, don't be afraid, I won't hit you, you take it as it comes." He was a happy chappie.'

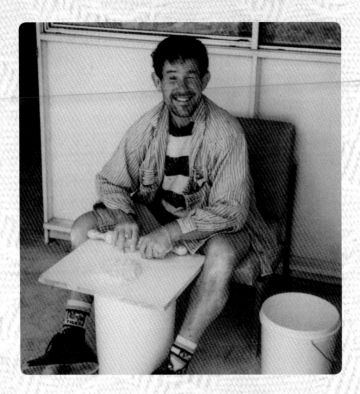

Ralph Dawson recycling clay at
Network Q, circa 1995. (Courtesy of Jan
Sharp, private collection)

As Ralph grew older he wanted to leave Kew. In 2006, after 41 years, he was relocated into a community residential unit. He was thrilled to have his own room which could be locked, 'I'm very happy here … I've got my keys and my own bedroom … No more sharing.'

Ralph returns to Kew regularly, as he works at VATMI, which is located on the periphery of the institution's grounds. He eagerly reports on the gradual dismantling of the Cottages and the construction of the new housing estate. Although he never wants to live at the institution again, he sometimes misses the independence of walking around his old neighbourhood and dropping in for a coffee and a chat with friends in other units.

John Goddard[10]

In 1956, John Goddard was born in rural Victoria. From an early age, he lived in special care facilities run by the Spastic Society of Victoria. At the age of nine John was admitted to Kew.

John had virtually no contact with his family. He did, however, forge long-time friendships with two volunteers, Lois Lockwood and Judy Osborne. John remarked that he was lucky to have friends like Lois and Judy who also invited him to be part of their own family celebrations. As we flipped through his photo album we came to a picture of Lois's husband Graham. John shouted 'Get your hands off my wife!' This was a mutual joke shared between John and Graham. John also expressed excitement about the birth

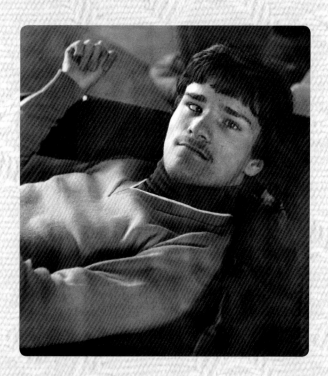

John Goddard at Kew Cottages, circa 1977. (Courtesy of Kew Residential Services, Department of Human Services, Victoria)

of Judy's grandson and forthrightly stated, 'You were going to bring the baby down Jude.'

John liked being employed in the Workshop, 'I used to do pegs and mops ... Spin, spin, cut the mops up, little mops.' He also earned money as a salesman, 'I used to sell the papers ... [and] get money for the papers I sold.'

Most of the time, John did not mind the communal nature of life at Kew. However, he despised living in Unit 21, where he spent a year. 'I didn't like it ... It was awful and I didn't like the food in the kitchen.' John was happy when he moved to Unit 25, declaring 'Twenty-five's better.'

John preferred living in a single bedroom as it offered privacy and personal space to listen to his music and watch television programs of his choosing. His favourite programs included, 'Wheel of Fortune', 'Countdown' and 'Big Brother'. John recalled that he especially loved to watch Essendon play matches during the footy season even when 'they did not win'. He is a true fan.

John was a regular guest at offsite social events run by Club Wild where he played musical instruments, danced and sang to his heart's content. 'I've been going to Club Wild ... Every month we go there ... sit up near the band.' On occasion, he even performed, 'I used to go up and sing with the man.'

John is one of the last remaining residents living at Kew. After 43 years in the institution, he will be relocated into an onsite community residential unit. When I asked if he was looking forward to moving he simply answered 'Yeah.'

Andrew Ledwidge[11]

In 1965, at the age of four, Andrew Ledwidge went to Kew Cottages for respite care. During his stay, Andrew celebrated his fifth birthday. Only a month after being discharged, he was re-admitted to the Cottages and he remained there for the next 41 years.

Even though he is a very private man, Andrew shared memories of people and events that were special to him. Some of these were treasured recollections of family life before living at Kew, 'I watched Dad be a gardener, at Kilmore, mowing the grass … a Victa mower, a black one.' He also remembered going on family outings 'my parents had the Wolseley at Kilmore, the Wolseley beetle, a brown Wolseley beetle.'

When he arrived at the Cottages, Andrew lived in Wilma Keller's children's ward. He recalled that in his early years, his favourite activities were playing with toys and musical instruments at occupational therapy (OT) sessions, 'at OT there was a plastic accordion, a circle one, red one'.

Andrew also remembered music being a part of the education program at the Special School where teacher 'John Doherty … [was] playing the piano and singing "Waltzing Matilda" … [and] "Work-

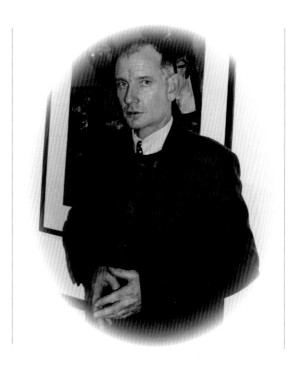

Andrew Ledwidge pictured in front of his artwork at a public exhibition, 2000. (Courtesy of Kew Residential Services, Department of Human Services, Victoria)

ing on the Railroad"'. As an adult, Andrew's musical interests and talents led to his participation in concerts. On one occasion he even composed and performed a song, 'Car Wash Blues', as part of the World Congress for Inclusion International which was held in Melbourne in 2003.

Each year, Andrew looked forward to Kew's Annual Fete, a festive occasion where residents mingled with crowds of people from the institution and the general community. Andrew remarked that he loved to ride on the 'old ghost train'. He also saved some of his money so he could buy specialty items off the stalls including, 'a tape-deck … cameras … ice creams [and] fairy floss'.

Andrew was unhappy when transferred from Unit 26/27 to live in the House Hostel. He voiced his protests 'I didn't like it … I talked to the social worker … [I said] "Move back to 26".' He felt that his request was not being heard and ran away in order to be taken seriously. Andrew's campaign was successful, and he was sent back to 26/27.

In 2006, Andrew was relocated into a community residential unit with four of his close friends. Initially, Andrew often asked when he could go back to live at Kew. During our first interview he said to the house manager, 'Talk to Peter Sabin, I want to move back to Kew … To *live* there.' Despite knowing that the institution was closing, Andrew wanted to return to a familiar haunt. However he has gradually settled comfortably into his new home, 'I like it better here.'

Donald Starick[12]

In 1968, at the age of six, Donald Starick was admitted to Kew Cottages. Previously, Donald had lived at home with his family in rural Victoria and had spent three months in a State institution known as Pleasant Creek in Stawell.

When Donald arrived at Kew he was placed in Ward 33 alongside children of his own age. At first, he found it difficult to settle and often cried out for his mother. He said that it was 'hard'. At the

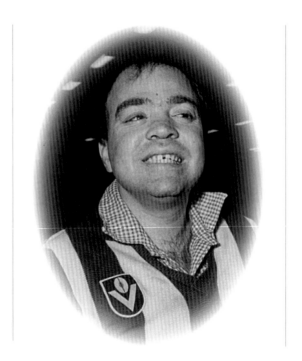

Kangaroos fan, Donald Starick, circa 1990. (Courtesy of Kew Residential Services, Department of Human Services, Victoria)

age of eight, Donald moved to the 'Schoolboys Ward'. As the years went by, he gradually acclimatised. Life at Kew was 'Alright.'

Many of Donald's memories were associated with attending life skills programs. He loved trips into community places such as shopping centres, 'Bus Friday … Shopping … buy clothes.' Some of his favourite activities involved music, dance and cookery. He preferred to sing nursery rhymes and Christmas carols, 'Music, la-la-la-la'.

Like a great number of other Kew residents Donald was keen on football. He is one of the Kangaroos most ardent fans. At Kew, Donald was fortunate to meet a few football players who visited residents on special occasions. He was also taken to matches by staff members who worked in his day program.

Donald enjoyed walking around the Kew grounds. In the years before he left Kew, each evening he would collect the Day Reports from many units and deliver them by torchlight to the Administration building, 'Report ... in Admin ... night ... torch.' On arrival, he would enjoy a coffee and a chat with staff members 'Jim ... [and] Barry'.

Donald was lucky as his family often wrote, phoned, visited and had him home for holidays. Family connections were very special to Donald and one of his program activities involves writing home to his mother, 'Write letters Mum'. Donald still gauges time by special occasions and planned visits to his family, 'Go home Easter'.

In May 1998, Donald was seriously injured after falling through the window of his first floor bedroom. No one knows how this happened, whether it was an accident or someone intentionally pushed him. 'Unit one ... Little window ... Man ... Ambulance ... Doctor ... Hospital'. Donald spent months recuperating in St Vincent's Hospital and the Hospital Unit at Kew. Even in 2007, the cause of his fall still remained a mystery.

In 2006, Donald moved into a community residential unit. After 38 years of living in institutional care he adjusted to community life with relative ease. Although he was used to residing at Kew, Donald prefers living a 'happy' life in his new home.

Nick Konstantaras[13]

Nick Konstantaras was born in 1960. He was nine years of age when he went to live at Kew Cottages. For 35 years, Nick progressed through various wards and units at Kew. When I asked if he liked living in the dormitories he replied, 'Yeah, you been before? ... You've seen them? ... They're big mate!'

Nick was a keen worker and a central figure at the carwash in Network Q and VATMI. 'I cleaned cars ... I wash the whole lot.' Nick used his earnings to buy special items from the onsite kiosk and shops at Kew Junction, 'I buy Coke ... pies and chicken.'

When unusual activities were going on at Kew, Nick always

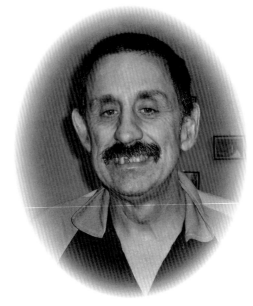

Nick Konstantaras, circa 2006.
(Courtesy of Nick Konstantaras, private
collection)

wanted to be part of the action. During a couple of strikes, staff and union members organised picket lines at the front entrance of the Cottages. Although residents were strictly forbidden from going near the picket area, Nick recalled his efforts to talk to the picketers, keeping them company and participating in the protests, 'Paul Wheatley, he was there too … Paul was in the strike … I'd say "Get lost, don't come back in Kew."' Nick was sent away by striking workers who had to adhere to established protocols.

Nick was one of the main people featured in a documentary film called *Exit Q*. This film recorded the experiences of a small number of residents who lived at Kew. It also documented the journey of three residents, including Nick, who were relocating away from the Cottages and into community housing.

The film makers wanted the final product to be truly collaborative and positive relationships were formed between production staff and residents. Nick spoke fondly of many people in the production team, particularly its producer, Phil Heuzenroeder, 'Oh Phil's a good man.' Nick was proud of his role in making the documentary, 'I did a good job.' He was also excited about having attended the film's premiere, 'I was dressed up and I went to a party.'

Nick recalled that one of the major disadvantages of living at Kew was the destruction of personal property. His television set was intentionally destroyed by a fellow resident. 'Peter Small smashed my TV.' This was a major blow for Nick as watching television was one of his favourite pastimes. Although there was a communal television set in the lounge room, Nick lost the freedom to enjoy programs of his own choosing in the privacy of his bedroom.

In 2004, Nick moved into a community residential unit. He was happy to leave Kew Cottages. When I asked Nick about his new house he jokingly replied, 'Well Blackburn's dreadful!' Then he laughingly declared, 'No Blackburn's alright!'

James Barry Woods[14]

James Barry Woods was born on 27 September 1934. He grew up in a Melbourne suburb with his parents and three siblings. James attended school until the age of 14, 'I was a student … I went to … the State school.' During this time James received private tuition and won a prize for 'mental arithmetic'.

When he completed school, James remained at home doing odd jobs. At the age of 32, after a disagreement with his parents, James fled from his home and into the street. He accidentally knocked over a child who was walking on the footpath and ran out into oncoming traffic, 'I had a car accident … I was just hit and knocked by a car.' The driver of the car and mother of the child lodged official complaints with police.

This episode resulted in James' admission to Royal Park Psychiatric Hospital. In 1966, he was transferred to Mont Park, then Sunbury Training Centre, 'I went to Sunbury … 24 years in there, that's true.' James explained that when Sunbury closed, 'I had to go to Kew.'

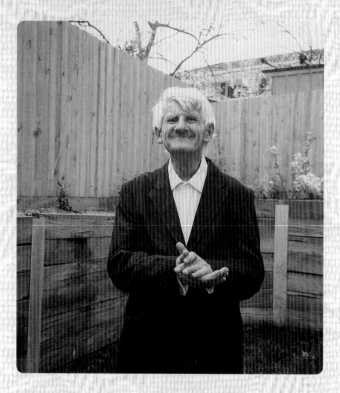

James Barry Woods at his community
residential unit, 2006. (Courtesy of
James Barry Woods, private collection)

On his first day at Kew, James lashed out at staff demanding to
be returned to Sunbury. However within days he had settled. He
particularly liked living in Unit 26/27, 'I used to be in 26 ... it was
a good ward.' He stated that Kew staff taught him about respecting
other people, 'you've got to do the right thing ... treat people with
respect'. This lesson appeared to be directly related to the staff-resident relationship as James further explained that 'respect' meant,
'doing what they ask you, and to do what you're told.'

James was considered by staff to be 'a social butterfly'. He loved
to walk around the grounds at Kew, visiting people, 'I made friends
at Kew ... We used to go for walks to the kiosk ... I used to go to
19 for a cup of tea.' James noted that he regularly met staff member

Peter Sabin, 'he's a good man, he gave me dry biscuits, Saladas.'

Although James claimed to be generally happy at Kew, he was also the victim of violence. On one occasion, a fellow resident attacked James, kicking him several times. Nearby staff stopped the attack. The police were called in to deal with the situation and were abused by the offender who was subsequently placed under close supervision for the remainder of the day. James was sent to the Hospital Unit for overnight observation.

In 2005, James was relocated into a community residential unit. He said, 'I had to come to Mitcham, Peter Sabin told me … because Kew was closing down.' Although he had moved several times before, James found it difficult to settle at first. At Mitcham, James demanded to be returned to Kew. However, over the weeks and months he grew to enjoy his new life in the community. In 2006, he stated, 'Mitcham's a good place.'

CHAPTER 7

'Chattel Slaves'?

*I was so happy to get to work, I couldn't stay
in the bloody ward at Kew, I couldn't stay
there any longer ... I like staying at work all
the time, to get away, just to get away from
the staff.*

Clare Turner, resident, 5 August 2005

From its earliest days, Kew Cottages attempted to provide opportunities for people with intellectual disability to develop skills
through education and training. Over the decades various transfor-
mations took place in the administration of education and training
at the Cottages, but on the whole programs were similar in content.
Up until the mid-1950s, these consisted of a blend of traditional
formal education and vocational training. With the introduction of
occupational therapy at the Cottages in the mid-1950s, the life skills'
programs burgeoned. Various facilities were created to increase
residents' access to these programs, but with limited staffing and
resources only a minority of residents enjoyed these services. A large
number of residents were also trained in the wards and were used as
additional labour to supplement the inadequate workforce. 'Resident

workers' were an invaluable 'commodity' in the daily operation of the institution as they were mostly unpaid. In 1937, Melbourne's *Truth* newspaper, a sensationalist weekly publication, condemned the use of 'resident workers' as an exploitative institutional practice; branding them as 'little better than chattel slaves'.[1] However, many residents enjoyed being part of an elite group, and garnered privileges that were unavailable to non-workers.

On 20 February 1929, the first Education Department school was opened at Kew Cottages. Teacher in charge, Frank Graham and his assistant, Olive Forrington, were responsible for instructing 34 children in a former dining area located in the male section of the institution.[2] This figure represented around seven per cent of residents living at the Cottages. Ted Rowe recalled being a pupil:

CORINNE Did you go to school?

TED Oh yes, had to go to school ... five days [a week].

CORINNE And were there lots of people at the school or was it just a small group?

TED Oh no, it was a big group. They used mostly the dining room for schools because [they] haven't got any other place ... [we did] woodwork and all of that ... I learned to read. Oh yes, had to learn that if I was going to go out, get a job.[3]

Clearly, during the 1920s and '30s education was promoted as a vehicle for some residents to move away from the institution and into mainstream Australian society. However, the testimony of resident interviewees from the 1950s did not mirror this viewpoint.

Only a minority of residents benefited from official education at Kew. The average rate of pupils who attended the school from the late 1920s was between five to 10 per cent of the total population. A major exception to this trend was in the late 1930s when this figure reached approximately 20 per cent. In 1937, the total population of Kew Cottages was 500. This figure fell to 276, in 1938, primarily through the transfer of 'more promising' residents to alternate State training facilities such as Janefield. Transfers impacted upon the percentage rate of residents attending education programs. However, this figure gradually reduced throughout the 1940s, when Kew accepted increasing numbers of residents. By 1950, 505 residents lived onsite. The number of students attending the school was on average 55.[4] According to teacher, Kay McCulloch, from 1938–58 there were no female students.[5] This was due to the external transfer of many female residents who were suitable for education to Janefield. Other female residents who had remained at the Cottages had the capacity to benefit from education, but were considered ineligible due to reasons such as age, level of disability or institutional work commitments.[6]

Evelyn Richards worked as a schoolteacher at Kew from 1940–44. Although dissatisfied with the poor condition of most Kew buildings, she was relatively content with school facilities, 'The main school was one of the better buildings. It had one very large school room, where perhaps three teachers taught. There was a small room for conveniences, and ... a small room where the head teacher ... had an office.'[7] Evelyn recalled that the official regulation of school attendance between five and 16 years of age was sometimes overlooked at the Cottages. She noted that a few adults aged in their early 20s were in attendance as they displayed the greatest potential for advancement.

With limited staff and resources at the school, some residents attended external classes and programs. For example, trade classes were offered by Collingwood Technical School.[8] This group of residents was highly advantaged as in this period most others were locked inside wards. The relationship between Collingwood and Kew continued over the years with many residents attending a broad range of programs and classes in 2007.

Aside from Ted Rowe, all of the interviewees who attended school at Kew did so in the 1950s–70s. In the 1960s and '70s, Andrew Ledwidge attended the Special School. He received lessons taught at other State schools, such as writing and art, but mostly enjoyed music:

ANDREW There was singing ... playing the piano, and singing.

CORINNE Who would play the piano?

ANDREW Mr Doherty, John Doherty.

CORINNE Can you remember any of the songs he played?

ANDREW 'Waltzing Matilda' ... [and] 'Working on the Railway'.[9]

Raymond Bouker also had memories of singing at the piano, with 'This Old Man' a favourite, 'I liked that one ... "This Old Man" ... It went up to 10!'[10] It was not surprising that Raymond was fond of this song as he had a penchant for numbers. 'Learning sums' was one of his preferred lessons. Another feature of school life that Andrew and Raymond enjoyed was drinking small cartons of milk at morning tea time. Andrew recalled, 'we used to have triangle milk cartons ... with straws ... from the Head Kitchen'.[11] Raymond was the milk monitor for his class, 'I used to go up to the kitchen, bring ... cartons of milk ... all by myself.'[12] Pupils were fortunate in being allocated milk for morning tea; this was an additional nutritional supplement that was unavailable in the wards.

From the 1950s, various health and medical experts were appointed at Kew. New forms of education and training were introduced in response to overseas and local influences. In 1953, Scottish psychiatrist Maxwell Jones published the influential *Therapeutic Community* which advocated a more multidisciplinary and inclusive approach to institutional care.[13] Reforms were also implemented by Eric Cunningham Dax and the Mental Hygiene Authority. From 1952 specialist groups of health professionals were employed at Kew to cater for the education and training needs of residents. Social workers were crucial in facilitating residents' access to classes within and outside of the institution. Other professional staff included occupational, physio, speech and music therapists. The 1950s saw a growth in life skills programs that eventually became an inherent part of life at Kew.

Occupational therapists made a significant contribution to

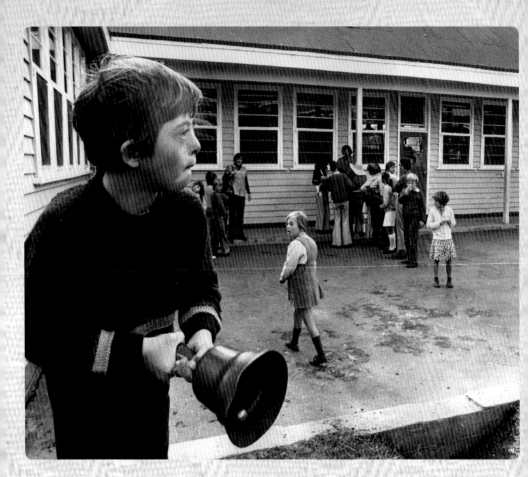

Students at the Special School, Kew Cottages, 1975. (Courtesy of *The Age* Archives/*The Age*, Melbourne)

training residents at the Cottages. In 1955 the Occupational Therapy (OT) Centre was officially opened through funds contributed by the Lions Club and Pamplin-Green bequest. The emphasis on training was to 'enable patients to be useful members of the institution community' and to prepare them for possible relocation to more advanced training centres.[14] OT sessions provided practical skills development for residents of varying ages and abilities. From 1960–70, around a fifth of residents were recipients of activities run by OT.[15] These figures were representative of the levels of service provided for residents until the 1980s.

Occupational therapists offered instruction in three distinct areas: the kindergarten, which catered for children aged five to 10 years, an intermediate class and pre-vocational Workshop.[16] Alongside therapy sessions, activities at the centre included sewing, cookery, laundry, housework, painting, typewriting and film screenings.[17] OT was an important forum for therapists to teach residents motor and communication skills, while imparting acceptable forms of personal and social behaviour. These skills were essential from the 1960s as greater interaction was fostered between residents and people living in mainstream society. Many staff understood that if positive relationships were to be formed then residents needed to adhere to social mores.

It was evident that some childhood activities at Kew had a lasting impact on residents' lives. Although some therapies, such as play and music therapy, may have appeared to be more recreational than educational, there was a sound basis for running such programs. In play therapy, residents were encouraged to use toys and playtime as a form of expression and communication. By closely supervising residents at play, therapists were able to assess and support them according to individual needs.[18] Residents, such as Andrew Ledwidge, looked forward to participating in playtime and music. Whenever he discussed OT, Andrew always recalled his delight in imagining programs being aired on a pretend television set: 'A wooden one with a wide screen … [I'd] see if there's any picture on the white Perspex screen.'[19] Andrew's adult interests in music and collecting model and toy aeroplanes, was reflected at time spent at OT:

CORINNE What else did you play with, besides the television box?

ANDREW The aeroplane, the bi-plane, plastic bi-plane, a red one.

CORINNE Is that where you got interested in planes?

ANDREW Yes, yes.

CORINNE Anything else, were there any music boxes, or were they somewhere else, not OT?

ANDREW Yes at OT it was, a plastic accordion …

CORINNE And would you play with that?

ANDREW Yes, yes.[20]

In 2006, when Andrew moved to a community residential unit he proudly displayed his aeroplane collection and musical instruments in his bedroom. On several occasions when I visited Andrew, he invited me to see his collection and played music on his guitar, harmonica and Italian made, wooden accordion.

The OT Workshop was pivotal in providing independent living skills and vocational training for eligible residents. Workshop

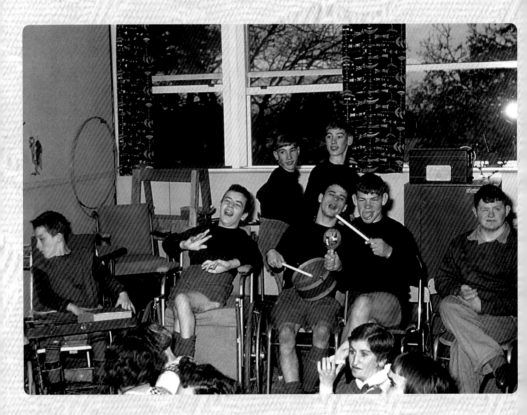

Residents participating in a percussion band at Kew, 1960s. (Courtesy of Kew Cottages Historical Society)

activities ranged from making pegs, mops, baskets and poppies for Remembrance Day to compiling safe sex kits, cutlery for airlines and packing boxes with goods such as plastic drink bottles. John Goddard enjoyed going to the Workshop:

JOHN   I used to do pegs and mops.

CORINNE   What did you do with mops?

JOHN   Spin, spin, cut the mops up, little mops.

CORINNE   So you'd cut the mop. Would you put them in packages?

JOHN   Yeah.[21]

Wendy Pennycuick worked in a different area:

CORINNE   And what sorts of things did you do at Workshop?

WENDY   Boxes, oh beads and boxes.

CORINNE   And would you get paid for that?

WENDY   Yes ... every week, every Friday.[22]

The OT Workshop provided a stimulating environment where residents learned new skills. Some sessions, such as classes on housekeeping, were education-based programs, while others were industrial activities where residents were paid a nominal wage for their labour.

One of the main benefits for OT Workshop attendees was the chance to socialise with people from other units. Clare Turner, who worked packing rubbish bags, brackets and serviettes, valued the company of Workshop colleagues. She described work as 'fun, fun, real fun'.[23] Clare did not want to return to her unit at the end of a working day, 'Doing all this work and all the people you talked ... I was so happy to get to work ... I don't feel like, feel like going home [to the unit]. I think when it's time to go home I said: "Oh no, do I have to go home?"'[24]

The OT Workshop closed in the late 1980s. For years afterwards, a few residents continued to arrive for work each morning. Administrative officer, Jan Sharp, was saddened and somewhat angered by the sight of these residents:

> The clients were still coming down at nine o'clock. They still hadn't got out of the habit of it and they found them nothing to do in its place. Now that, I think, is disgusting. I thought it at the time and I haven't changed my opinion. You don't take something away without putting something as good or better in its place.[25]

Although a small group of residents milled around the closed Workshop, many others were given alternate placements at day programs and at Network Q, a sheltered workshop located at Kew Cottages. These new programs and activities enabled residents to develop existing skills and to enjoy new environments and opportunities.

From the 1950s to the '70s, some nursing and OT staff offered activity programs in the wards for residents who were unable to access regular sessions elsewhere. Many of these programs were intended to provide practical training for residents in daily care and mobility. Occupational therapist, Saral Nathaniel, stated that in one unit, 'The clients all had cerebral palsy, most of them were on wheelchairs … [we worked] in the unit … providing activities such as playing with the balls, music and the handicraft and art.'[26] Similarly, a few nurses taught residents about personal care. Maria Kraushofer relied upon institutional behaviours associated with routine and repetition to teach independent living skills in her ward:

> we put a lot of emphasis on the routine, repeat, repeat, repeat until it was taught. And they knew what was happening. The minute we changed something we had to make sure that every single staff knew it was changed. Then we started slowly building on that change again and continuing that change until they got that. That's how we achieved the toileting, that's how we got them after meals to wash their faces, that's how we achieved that if they soiled themselves they would go and clean themselves.[27]

In 1977, four education centres, funded by the Minus Children Appeal, were opened and staffed by Education Department

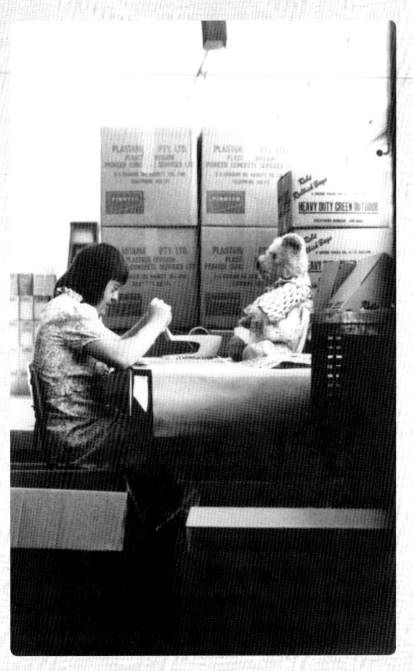

A female resident at the Workshop,
circa 1977. (Courtesy of Kew Cottages
Historical Society)

employees. Max Jackson was a teacher in the Geiger and Perkin centres from 1979–81. He explained, 'Our brief in fact was to provide "education" to residents who came up from the units on a daily basis.'[28] These facilities actively supported developmental and behavioural programs. Within four years of opening, it was evident that students' developmental needs would be more adequately met through a multidisciplinary approach.

In 1982, in response to this perceived need, Max was appointed Kew's first coordinator of programs. He was responsible for devising a strategy to combine the expertise of medical, health and education professionals, 'Throughout 1982–83 my brief was to establish these multidisciplinary teams … I think from memory there were about 120 staff altogether. We decided we'd create eight teams with two operating out of each of the Minus Children's buildings.'[29] A variety of programs were offered ranging from human relations to art, physical education to sensory-motor activities. Alma Adams worked as a team leader in Hamer, 'I've got some extraordinarily happy memories of working in the Hamer Centre in Kew. I've got memories of taking people on boating trips to the Gippsland Lakes. Little memories of the guys running across from Unit 31, with their faces lighting up because they were going to be in Mick Ellis's [phys ed] program and they really enjoyed it.'[30] Alma also recalled that, like previous OT programs, centre staff wanted to foster positive relationships with people working in the units:

> One of the things that a number of us were very keen on was, rather than just having a multidisciplinary team around the centres and the unit staff in units, we wanted to try and pull the whole thing together. So 'centre' staff would work in the units in the early morning to increase the staff ratio and enable more individualisation.[31]

Ralph Dawson attended the Perkin Centre to participate in a range of activities including art classes that involved painting and the production of ceramic ware:

RALPH I worked in Perkins. I had to wear a mask, put a mask on, and soak all the clay. I was pretty good at doing that. I'd soak

the clay, put it in the bucket, start again, brush some more ...
I was pretty good at filling the bucket up to the top. You make
slip out of it.

CORINNE And what's slip?

RALPH To make pottery.[32]

At various times from the late 1970s to 2007, other education and
training facilities complemented the activities offered at the Minus
Children's buildings. Some facilities included the Special School, Kew
Adult Training Support Service and Kew Day Programs. During this
period efforts were made to provide most residents with programs or
work at Kew.

Education and training initiatives at Kew were supported by
many parents who believed that the quality of life for residents was
greatly enhanced through program and work activities. In 1995,
the continual reduction in programs available for residents was a
major contributor to the Parents' Association suing the Victorian
Government. Association member, Hilda Logan, stated:

> when the Kennett Government came in, we had 150 program staff,
> by the time they went out we had 40. We never ever had enough
> program staff to give everybody a full program. A few of them
> [residents] that worked in Network Q might have got 30 hours a
> week, or something like that, but others were only getting two hours
> a week, not a day, a week.[33]

The potential of day programs to improve the lives of residents was
noted by Andrew Slevin, who worked in the Kew Day Program
service from 1999 until its closure in 2006:

> KDP as it was known, was a place where residents were assisted to
> actively engage in communication via music, song, dance, art and
> craft and sports games. This provided the residents stimulation in
> what was sometimes a stale environment.[34]

Andrew argued that supplying ample programs was not enough.
He believed that quality programming also relied upon a team of
motivated staff, 'Life at KDP was a challenge ... sadly due to a lack

of motivation life became dull for both the residents as well as the staff. KDP became a place of re-active instead of pro-active strategies and this held back the advancement of the residents' lives.[35] Andrew blamed the announced closure of Kew, and therefore KDP, as the primary source of staff discontent. This decision also resulted in increasing numbers of residents attending external programs run by organisations such as Interact Australia, which had its origins in Kew Cottages.

Up until the 1950s, it would not have appeared unusual to classify much of the work being done by residents as 'therapy' or 'training'. 'Work therapy' was often prescribed for people living in 'mental institutions', including the farm at Kew Mental Hospital. However, some staff accounts, government and media reports clearly indicated that up until the 1970s, 'resident workers' at the Cottages were not being 'educated', but rather filled labour shortages that prevailed, particularly in the wards, kitchen and laundry.

'Resident workers' were often assigned to work in the central laundry that serviced both the Cottages and Mental Hospital. Ted Rowe recalled that mostly female residents worked in this area, but on occasion male workers were also seconded. Ted was happy to work in the laundry as it relieved the boredom of institutional life and gave him the rare opportunity to mix with female residents:

TED They come and asked us [to get the] sheets and that and fold them up, in the laundry, 'You can go down [to the] laundry and help them down there … So they cut that out after that because we were flirting with the girls.

CORINNE So you were flirting with the girls in the laundry?

TED Oh yeah, we had a good time … One of them wanted me to give them a kiss. I said 'Yeah when no one's watching you up there.'

CORINNE So you were trying to steal a kiss from the girls were you?

TED   Oh we tried to but we didn't.[36]

Residents worked hard and were required to wash, hang, iron and fold clothes and linen. Residents, such as Dolly Stainer, occasionally took advantage of their situation by smuggling in their personal clothing items and laundering them to the highest standard.[37] Dolly was proud of circumventing official institutional regulation. This behaviour also revealed her cleanliness and pride in her personal appearance.

With literally hundreds, and sometimes thousands, of meals to prepare each day, the central kitchen also relied upon resident labour to meet institutional demands. As mentioned in Chapter 5, up until the mid-1950s, the kitchen was often run by two to three official kitchen staff who were supported by a small group of around eight to 10 'resident workers'. For decades these workers were officially unpaid, but occasionally received gratuities for their efforts. In 1937, a public scandal erupted after a resident, identified as 'May K', was seriously injured while working in the kitchen. May was assisting staff when her hand became caught in a mincing machine, resulting in the loss of four fingers. An internal inquiry was held and findings concluded that May was responsible for causing the accident as she, 'had put her hand into the mincer without authority, and thus lost her fingers'.[38] The *Truth* newspaper berated institutional management and the Victorian Government for its finding and perceived exploitation of 'resident workers'. It suggested that institutional practice was to blame, not the resident:

> *"Truth"* puts it to the authorities that whether or not May was employed working the mincer, as certain people say, or was told not to go near it, as official version runs, the unfortunate child-woman should not have been working in the kitchen at all.[39]

Truth argued that the hundreds of residents working in State mental institutions were akin to slaves. Cunningham Dax agreed that 'resident workers' were being over-utilised. In the 1950s, he introduced measures to limit the use of 'resident workers' who lived in State facilities by recruiting a range of staff to assist in the day-today running of institutions. Despite staffing improvements, 'resident workers' remained essential labour at Kew as growing numbers of people were admitted. In 1952, when Cunningham Dax commenced work, there were 475 residents, by the time he left in 1969 this figure had risen to 948.[40] 'Resident workers' proved to be an indispensable necessity.

From early in the morning, residents who were considered to be 'higher functioning' and ambulant were often required to help staff in the wards. In the 1920s and '30s Ted Rowe had specific morning chores, 'we had our duties to do, to keep the dormitories all clean and everything and make the beds, make sure the beds were all clean, sheets on and everything ... they had no cleaners there, we had to do all the cleaning'.[41] When I asked if he helped other residents, particularly those with physical disabilities, he replied, 'No, they were in the other part, another dormitory, so we didn't have to worry about them.'[42]

The necessity for resident labour in the wards was notable during periods of overcrowding and in accommodation areas where residents with additional support needs were housed. Up until the 1970s, without this assistance, it would have been virtually impossible for staff to clean, feed and clothe residents. While some staff inculcated residents with the value of education through work and the virtue of 'helping fellow residents', others simply issued orders. Patty Rodgers was proud of supporting her fellow residents, 'I'd get Wendy out early in the morning ... I'd get her dressed.'[43] Wendy Pennycuick was grateful for Patty's assistance, 'Patty's a good helper.'[44] Raymond Bouker recalled that when he was a child living in Ward 33, 'I used to dress up the boys ... big and little.'[45] When I asked why he helped, he replied 'the staff told me'.[46] Patty and Raymond, along with many other residents, were vital in ensuring the smooth running of wards through facilitating morning activities such as showering, organising breakfast and preparing residents for school, work or day programs.

The majority of 'resident workers' received little recompense for their labour. Jeannette Hodgkinson, the daughter of superintendent

Wifrid Brady, recalled that when residents worked in their home, her mother gave them 'beautiful trays of morning and afternoon teas'.[47] She also paid 'resident workers' pocket money to purchase items at the kiosk. Lois Philmore, who worked in the Brady household, remembered, 'she paid me ... I did have my money, yes, in the dormitory ... In the tin.'[48] Residents' display of 'good behaviour' through work was also sometimes acknowledged by staff through personal attention and praise. When I interviewed Ralph Dawson, he wanted to make sure that his helpfulness was recorded. He said, 'I was a Mr Helpful ... I helped Donald Starick. I helped him out because Donald doesn't dress himself ... I have to help him out, put his socks on him ... Is that going on tape?'[49] Similarly, in 2007, Raymond Bouker frequently sought a pat on the back after folding and delivering washing to his fellow residents.

From the 1970s, domestic work was often classified as 'household chores' or 'training in independent living skills'. While in some respects these assertions may have appeared valid, historically, institutional work was not categorised in this manner. Until the 1960s, administrators tended to be more upfront in stating that 'resident workers' were a necessary part of institutional life, their exploitation was not hidden by the rhetoric of 'empowering individuals'.

While the use of unpaid labour was in many ways exploitative, it offered some residents benefits that were unavailable to non-workers. Female residents such as Katie Collins, Dolly Stainer and Lorna White, formed loving relationships through working with young residents in the Nursery Ward. They were responsible for cleaning, feeding and bathing children assigned to their care. Katie often referred to her charges as 'possum', while Dolly Stainer simply called them 'my babies'.[50] The role that Katie, Dolly and Lorna fulfilled, was highly valued, particularly by parents who visited Kew. Parent Joan Jones recalled, 'One day when I arrived I was met with a lovely sight. Dolly and Katy [sic] were sitting in the sun outside the Cottage and there on Dolly's knee was my little Richie, happy as Larry to be having a cuddle.'[51] A reciprocal relationship often existed between this group of 'resident workers' and children in the Nursery. Mutual affection was often exchanged, a prize highly valued in an institutional world where residents were habitually starved of meaningful interpersonal relationships.

A number of 'resident workers' made the most of their privileged position and enhanced their quality of life at the institution by taking advantage of opportunities as they arose. This was sometimes done in a covert manner, for example when Dolly surreptitiously cleaned personal items in the central laundry, or more openly when staff offered incentives, such as money, in return for favours or completing additional duties. Lois Philmore recalled, 'I used to clean Miss Lucas' car ... I washed it everywhere ... I did it myself, Miss Lucas got me to do it ... she paid me.'[52] When residents were allowed to roam more freely around the institution and its environs some consciously sought chances to make money. This allowed them to purchase special, personal items that many non-working residents could not afford such as hand-held radios and luxury toiletries.

In the mid-20th century, the introduction of industrial work at the Cottages resulted in a small group of residents being given a nominal wage for their labour. The OT Workshop ran on similar lines to a sheltered workshop, and was eventually replaced by Network Q, a more formal supported employment service. These facilities provided people with disabilities employment opportunities often unavailable in mainstream society. Pay levels at Kew were consistently far less than the basic wage, but allowed some residents to purchase personal items. Monetary payment was also an official recognition of the value of certain types of resident labour.

In the late 1980s, Network Q superseded the OT Workshop. It consolidated industrial activities that were being undertaken by some residents at Kew, and provided program and work opportunities. Residents were able to earn a small income at Network Q through employment in areas such as gardening, cleaning, catering, art, office work and car washing. Although much work was done onsite, some residents were sent into the community, for example to clean private residences. Nick Konstantaras was excited when recalling his work at the car wash:

CORINNE Did you ever work at the car wash?

NICK Yeah I did.

CORINNE What did you do?

NICK I cleaned cars, outside, the windows.

CORINNE You cleaned cars outside, you cleaned the windows?

NICK Do you see me at the car did you?

CORINNE I did, I've seen you at the car wash.

NICK Yeah I wash the whole lot that's all.

CORINNE You washed the whole lot?

NICK Yeah.

CORINNE Inside and out? Would you do it a lot?

NICK Yeah, five, a lot, that's all.

CORINNE Would you do it for five days or five cars?

NICK Five [days].[53]

Andrew Ledwidge worked alongside Nick. Andrew preferred washing cars to other work available at Kew as it paid more money.[54] In 2005, when Network Q merged with VATMI industries, a not-for-profit company employing people with disabilities, 'resident workers' were relocated to VATMI's new premises on the perimeter of the Cottages in Hutchinson Drive. When the car wash service was forced to close in 2007 due to water restrictions caused by drought, Andrew and Nick were reassigned to the packaging area. Although Andrew was resigned to the temporary closure, he anxiously waits for rain so that he can return to his favourite job, cleaning cars and buses.

When deinstitutionalisation initiatives were introduced in the 1980s, 'resident workers' were considered to be the most suitable candidates for relocation. The skills that many 'resident workers' learned equipped them to find employment in the mainstream community. Patrick Reed was a perfect example, 'I started to work in the Stores of Kew Cottages and then I learned to work over in the Workshop, fixing little cars and things.'[55]

Patrick thoroughly enjoyed being able to move around the Cottages and to meet a variety of people on his travels. One of Patrick's jobs when he moved away from Kew was working at Rojo Panel Beaters where his mechanical skills were put to use, 'at Rojo Panel, [I] used to do clutches, put clutches in there too, because they heard about Kew when I was there, and they came around and asked me would I like to work there.'[56] Patrick was fortunate in securing work in an occupation that he enjoyed.

Some staff were concerned that as 'resident workers' moved away from Kew their sense of purpose and self-identity would diminish. John Wakefield believed that Patrick Reed suffered. 'Paddy's problem was that he had dignity, respect and a position as a "working boy". Nowadays he's looking for that, and I don't think he's getting it.'[57] There was no denying that workers such as Patrick held high status positions among residents in the institutional hierarchy. Despite this, when he resided at Kew, Patrick was constantly running away. After leaving the Cottages Patrick lived independently in the community. Although he struggled with many issues, particularly loneliness, he believed that the benefits of living in the general community far outweighed those associated with life as a 'resident worker' at Kew. When I asked Patrick whether he was content to leave Kew he answered, 'Ooh, quite happy ... I had freedom.'[58]

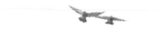

CHAPTER 8

Happy Memories?

I witnessed beautiful things there [at Kew]. I remember going past the kitchen door of one of those old-fashioned places one day and somebody had knocked over a chair. They had a kiddie in there who was about eight or nine ... sitting on the floor but he was very disabled physically. He reacted so badly to this chair being knocked over, and one of the little Down Syndrome kids ran over to a big pile of clean white nappies and took one off and went over and got down alongside him and dabbed his eyes. It was so beautiful.

Reverend James Scannell, Catholic priest assigned to Kew, 13 December 2006

Life was tough for Kew Cottages' residents who were isolated from society in a highly impersonal world. In his study *Asylums*, Erving Goffman argued that facilities like Kew relied upon regimented and often dehumanising mechanisms to operate in an efficient manner.[1] This was certainly evident at the Cottages where schedules dominated individual needs and interpersonal relationships. However, there were many people associated with Kew who tried to compensate for the failings of the institution. Additional care and support were provided by a range of people including residents, staff, parents and volunteers. Their assistance was above and beyond that offered by successive Victorian Governments. The contribution of these people varied and included establishing meaningful personal relationships, assisting in program delivery, organising social activities and holding fundraising events. Compassion, dedication and humanity have been noteworthy in Kew's history.

For many residents the most positive aspect of life at Kew was the relationships forged with others at the institution. These relationships were sometimes a substitute for a lack of familial contact and were an important survival mechanism. Generally, relationships formed between residents were based upon notions of companionship. However, in some cases meaningful romantic bonds and sexual partnerships also existed. Personal relationships enabled some residents to enjoy intimate moments where they communicated and shared desires, experiences and opinions about institutional life. When recording sessions with resident interviewees, I welcomed the involvement of partners, friends and housemates. During our conversations it was enlightening to witness the interaction between some residents who joked around, prompted memories and even finished one another's sentences. These sessions brought to the fore the deep understanding, camaraderie and mutual concern shared between some residents.

Many residents highly valued their friendships with other residents at Kew. This was notable when they spoke about the loss, injury or illness of someone with whom they were close. Ralph Dawson described his response to the news that his friend, Donald Starick, fell from his first floor bedroom window:

RALPH   He fell out the window, and landed on the concrete floor, outside, he was in a bad way ... He went to St Vincent's Hospital and had four operations on him.

CORINNE   And how did you feel when you found out he'd been hurt?

RALPH   I burst in tears, I was very upset.

CORINNE   Did you go and see him?

RALPH   Yes I did, he was in Smorgon (Hospital Unit at Kew).

CORINNE   Was that before or after he went to St Vincent's?

RALPH   When he came back … He was in a bad way, he had pins in his legs.[2]

Ralph and Donald have been friends since their childhood days at Kew. They have maintained their friendship even when sometimes living in separate units. They are now delighted to live together in a community residential unit.

Throughout its history, sexual and romantic relationships existed among residents at Kew, many surreptitiously. These relationships were mostly frowned upon by staff who considered sexual contact to be problematic. Staff concern was evident in their vigi-

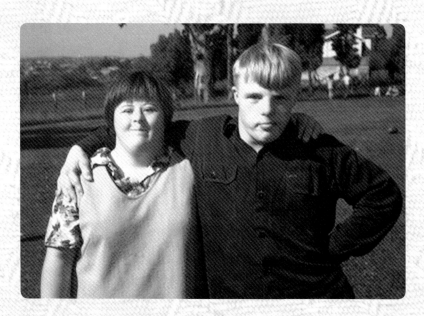

Kew residents, 1970s. (Courtesy of Kew
Cottages Historical Society)

lance to maintain the gender division until the 1960s. From the 1970s, Kew Cottages operated according to the popular principles of normalisation, advocacy and citizen rights. An inherent element of these philosophies was acknowledging that residents had a right to be sexual beings. The official model of sexuality and sexual expression which prevailed at Kew from this time onwards adhered to social mores that existed in Australian society. These reflected ideas of monogamy and the creation of 'safe' partnerships. Some residents who were considered to be sexually active were sent to human relations programs or were advised individually by staff.

The importance of romantic and sexual partnerships to some residents was highlighted when residents moved away from the Cottages. When deinstitutionalisation was introduced, some couples who had been together for years were being physically separated. This was the case for Kew residents Heather and Kevin. In a musical written for the World Congress for Inclusion International, staff at Northern Metropolitan TAFE worked with Heather to compose a song that expressed the loss that she and Kevin felt when he was relocated from Kew. Her song related to the musical's theme about separation through hospitalisation, but was in fact based upon the loss and loneliness experienced by her and Kevin. The song was titled 'I Came Back' and included the following:

> He was crying today because I went away
> He was scared I went away
> Scared I wouldn't come back
> But I did come back
> I caught the bus back to my lover.[3]

Partnerships, such as Heather and Kevin's, were meaningful and allowed residents to find solace in a place that was dominated by adversity.

Despite the efforts of many staff to curb sexual activity, over half of the resident interviewees in this history spoke about having fulfilling relationships with boyfriends and/or girlfriends. This figure reflected the composition of the interview cohort who exercised a degree of independence within the institution and were teenagers when liberalised views of sexuality were introduced at Kew. Although same sex relationships existed at Kew, interviewees were unwilling to record their opinions on homosexuality at the institution or associated it with sexual abuse. When I raised the issue of homosexuality I was often quickly corrected by staff; these were same sex partnerships of convenience, not sexual preferences exercised by residents. The gender division was often 'blamed' for residents' homosexual tendencies. Staff member, Kurt Kraushofer argued, 'Residents, I don't consider them homosexuals because for many years they live two separate identities … males stayed over there and females over there.'[4] According to a study of sexuality and disability, this viewpoint emanated from ideas that people with disabilities were asexual or incapable of making informed choices.[5] This attitude was present among many staff and families at Kew. It was clearly evident in the responses given by a few residents that relationships with 'special friends' were also openly discouraged by some people at Kew:

CORINNE Who did you live with in 26/27?

STEVEN Oh, well with the boys.

CORINNE And did you have any special friends when you lived in 26/27?

STEVEN No, you don't do it![6]

Many resident interviewees spoke about meeting their partners and the pleasure that romantic and sexual relationships brought them. David Honner referred to two partnerships that he had at Kew:

CORINNE Was Lindy a friend, or a girlfriend?

DAVID A girlfriend.

CORINNE And did you go out with Lindy for a long time?

DAVID Yes.

CORINNE And how did you meet Lindy? Did she live near you, or did she live somewhere else?

DAVID   She was in my unit, in our unit.

CORINNE   And so you used to live together in a unit? Did you have your own rooms, or did you share?

DAVID   I had my own room. I was living with two boys.[7]

When his relationship ended with Lindy, David started seeing Monica, but they were separated when Monica was relocated into a community residential unit. David still sees Monica as the staff consider their partnership to be important and worthwhile. They sometimes meet at the cinema or a shopping centre, but now their visits are in the company of others. Nevertheless, David looks forward to these occasions 'I gave her a kiss last weekend.'[8] As in David and Monica's case, the continuation of romantic and sexual partnerships was often reliant upon staff willingness to actively support the ongoing relationships. In other circumstances people were relocated into community housing with their partners. Patty Rodgers was pleased to be able to continue her relationship, 'My boyfriend … [lives] with me … We've been girlfriends and boyfriends for a long time.'[9]

Affection between residents sometimes resulted in engagements. However, these unions were not always welcomed by families. Clare Turner was engaged to a fellow resident, but his family disapproved and the relationship was ended. Clare recalled, 'my boyfriend and me we was engaged, but his parents didn't want me because I was how I am now, disabled … in a wheelchair'.[10] Given the lack of personal space and privacy, staff and a few families were powerful in determining the types of relationships that many residents were able to enjoy. A small number of residents secretly met with one another in areas of the grounds that were hidden or rarely visited by people.

Some staff members forged positive professional and platonic relationships. Social worker, Fran van Brummelen, recalled that in the 1960s and '70s staff in the Nursery Ward knitted clothes for babies in their care. During this period, a charge nurse facilitated the donation of a Hammond organ to provide stimulus and entertainment for active male residents in his ward.[11] Manager, Jack Cotter, stated that particularly among the female nursing staff, 'there was some absolute angels'.[12] He admired the determination of women such as Margot Nacha, Millie Lucas and Wilma Keller, who doggedly fought for additional resources for their charges. They were not always successful, but constantly made demands to senior management. Jack noted, 'I mean to a manager, at times you'd feel they were a bit of a nuisance, because they were persistent, but it was all directed at looking after their kids.'[13] Prominent staff who were celebrated for their dedication were mostly concerned with residents in their direct care.

Some of the key staff members had a reputation for ruling with 'benevolent tyranny'.[14] They were not personally liked by colleagues, but were highly respected for their determination to enhance residents' lives. Nurse, Helen Wilson, worked alongside one woman who had a reputation for being difficult, 'this particular charge nurse, she was very tough, she was very stern, but overall she did a lot of new and exciting things for the residents, like take them on holidays to different places, [and] on day trips to different places'.[15] Residents included in these activities were those considered to be 'more attractive'; including those housed in the Nursery Ward, young children's wards or 'high functioning' people without challenging behaviours.

The devotion of some staff was revealed during times of industrial conflict. Staff and unions associated with Kew Cottages often resolved disputes without industrial action. This form of conflict resolution was preferred by all parties because of the possible negative implications for residents' welfare if staff were unable to attend to their daily needs. In the 1980s and '90s, a small number of strikes took place. Some people remained at Kew, as official skeleton staff and a few others covertly crossed picket lines by hiding in cars or using entry points away from the main road. Most strikingly, workers did not consider these staff members to be 'scab labour', understanding that they acted with the welfare of residents in mind rather than showing support for management. Parent, Hilda Logan, volunteered to work in her son's unit at Kew during the strikes. She was impressed by the efforts of staff to maintain the wellbeing of residents. She stated, 'They had put ... the name of everybody on their arm ... [with] Gentian Violet, which was a bit like mercurochrome ... to help anybody who was working in the unit.'[16] Hilda also remembered that a few staff 'came in the back gate and worked as volunteers'.[17]

A minority of staff members became friendly with individual residents and offered them special privileges not afforded to most people at Kew. These staff often allowed residents to become part of their familial and social worlds. They took them away from the institution for special occasions and sometimes even holidays. Permission from Kew management for this type of interaction was required. Patrick Reed was a welcome guest on a few occasions at a staff member's property located in Warrandyte.[18] He rode his bike from Kew in order to make these visits. Ruth Anghie sometimes took younger residents to her family home and provided them with special treats, recalling that her visitors valued their time away from institutional life.[19]

These friendly relationships were unusual, and often temporary, as staff moved around or away from the Cottages. Many residents enjoyed these close personal relationships with staff, but felt devastated when they lost such companionship. Ralph Dawson was very friendly with one staff member who took him on outings and holidays. When the person left Kew, contact gradually decreased and eventually stopped altogether. Ralph was upset, 'She don't like me no more. Why doesn't she call me or see me? She doesn't want to see me no more.'[20] This blurring of institutional and personal boundaries resulted in residents' expectations that the staff-resident relationship was in fact an enduring friendship. In a few rare cases this happened, but for most residents such 'friendships' were fleeting.

Volunteers who worked at Kew also established cordial relationships with many residents and made substantial improvements to the fabric of the institution. In the 20th century, a variety of individuals, community and welfare organisations were associated with the Cottages. From the 1930s, members the Mental Hospitals' Auxiliary visited the Cottages and on occasion took selected residents on outings into the community. The Auxiliary also funded practical works, such as the construction of a new school at Kew in 1952, to replace the previous building that was destroyed by fire.[21]

Chairman of the Mental Hygiene Authority, Eric Cunningham Dax, praised the first president of the Lions Club in Melbourne, Dudley Peck. He considered that Dudley was instrumental in facilitating improvements to the Cottages in the 1950s. In addition to co-funding the construction of the first onsite centre for occupational therapy, the Lions Club also helped to renovate dilapidated buildings. Cunningham Dax recalled that Dudley:

> mobilised a lot of people. They painted the whole of the outside of Kew Cottages and they did the roofs. There's a well known story about the man who went home with a lot of bars across his behind, as if he'd had corporal punishment or something. It turned out that he'd been painting the roofs of the Kew Cottages on a very hot day and he burnt his bottom on the corrugated iron.[22]

In the 1950s and '60s, people from mainstream society responded to Cunningham Dax's calls for the public to have greater involvement with institutions. In 1961, a formalisation of volunteerism at Kew resulted in the formation of the Visiting Services of Auxiliaries. In its heyday, in the 1970s and '80s, there were over 500 volunteers who assisted staff and residents at Kew.

From the 1960s procedures were introduced to inform, train and assign volunteers to work in specific areas of need. In 1974, Jan Sharp volunteered to work at Kew. Being a qualified swimming teacher, Jan worked closely with Kew staff to devise swimming programs that benefited residents:

> I was introduced to the Halliwick swim method which was an international method for teaching physically disabled … It's a 10 point program which is a sequence of getting people to balance, getting people's confidence up … I was very impressed with this and

I thought: 'I'll introduce it at Kew', which I did with huge success …
I set about getting more and more volunteers and in the end I had 60
volunteers a week helping me.[23]

Through her voluntary activities, staff realised Jan's potential and
subsequently she was paid to conduct the swimming program. This
was a service that was enjoyed by hundreds of residents, including
Steven Wears:

CORINNE   Did you enjoy swimming?

STEVEN   Yes … There was a hoist … It's very hard to get in.

CORINNE   And would someone help you?

STEVEN   Yes.[24]

Another area that developed from volunteer involvement was physical
education (phys ed). Robyn Cook started work as a volunteer in 1975.
Due to her experience as a phys ed teacher, she was asked by the
head physiotherapist to formulate programs for a range of residents
throughout the Cottages. Robyn was employed on a part-time basis,
but continued to volunteer. She basically worked full-time at the
Cottages until 1982. Robyn worked alongside other phys ed staff who
provided programs for a small group of residents through the Special
School and eventually the Minus Children's buildings. Robyn's
programs encouraged residents to become active. She recalled that
one of her primary goals was to help them overcome the 'Kew Shuffle',
a common term used to describe the walking movement of many
residents who forlornly shuffled around the institution:

We would get their heart beating and get their blood pumping. So
it was tumbling, rolling, climbing and music … In those days the
nurses who came were quite happy to join in and help, because you
couldn't have a whole unit by yourself, you'd *need to have help.*[25]

In the late 1970s, a Monday Night Club was established at Kew to
promote the involvement of residents in sport. Jan Sharp and Robyn
were leading organisers. Initially activities were centred around
swimming and gymnastics, but grew with the help of Kew staff and

volunteers, to include other sports such as athletics, basketball, soccer and tennis. Club activities were generally hosted at the Cottages, but external locations were sometimes sought when adequate facilities were unavailable. Jan stated that due to limited staffing and transportation, originally only independent residents were able to join the Club.[26] However, as support for the Club grew from staff and volunteers, gradually a small number of residents with higher support needs were able to attend. Throughout its 18-year operation, between 60 to 120 Kew residents regularly attended the Club.

Kew's Monday Night Club was significant as it was a major driving force in the development of Special Olympics in Victoria. In 1976, the secretary of the Mental Health Authority, Bill Woods, approached Kew's assistant director of nursing, Kurt Kraushofer, about starting the Special Olympics program in Australia. Bill's enthusiasm for this sporting event emanated from a trip to America where he witnessed first hand the advantages of Special Olympics for its participants.[27] According to Jan Sharp, in Victoria concerns were raised by professional educators about whether competitive sports were detrimental for people with intellectual disability. Many advocates of the Special Olympics disagreed with this viewpoint and were determined to prove otherwise. Jan stated, 'we were up against so many misinformed people. They weren't prepared to try, that's what gets me, I mean you can't say it won't work if you don't *try* it.'[28] Subsequently, inter-institution events, known as 'Fun Days', were held, mostly at Kew, which included swimming, athletics and gymnastics.

These sporting events were a resounding success. John Goddard enjoyed competing in swimming events and won a medal for his efforts.[29] Robyn recounted John's victory:

> I can remember him when he was at a Special Olympics swimming race, he was in front in a flotation race, where they lie on their back and kick like mad, and I was calling: 'Come on John' and he got to the end and I said: 'You *won*!' He said: 'Oh! I knew I could do it, Rob!'[30]

Kew Cottages produced several Special Olympians who travelled overseas and competed in a range of events. Sporting activities not only provided some residents with the opportunity to develop skills, but also enabled them to participate in events beyond the boundaries of the institution.

The success of special programs and events at Kew was partly due to the support of those families who took an active interest in the welfare of their relatives. As stated earlier, for some residents, families remained a constant in their lives. In 1957, a Parents' Association was formed. One hundred and thirty people attended the inaugural meeting. At its conclusion, 70 people signed up as official members.[31] From this time, a core group of parents, and sometimes other family members, facilitated a range of activities to support one another and enhance the lives of their relatives at Kew. These activities included public information sessions, special events, fundraising and pastoral care.

For residents, the most memorable activity offered by the Association was the Annual Fete run from 1961–2001. Resident, Andrew Ledwidge, recalled the excitement of seeing the tents and stalls being set up in the morning.[32] Another resident, Patty Rodgers, looked forward to collecting her boyfriend from his unit and walking around the festivities. She saved some of her money to buy items from various stalls:

CORINNE Did you buy anything from the fete?

PATTY Show-bag!

CORINNE Show-bags! That's my favourite part of fetes, it still is!

PATTY Yes!

CORINNE What would you buy to eat?

PATTY Hot dogs!

CORINNE What about fairy floss, did you like fairy floss?

PATTY Oh it's too messy.

CORINNE Too messy. Can you remember what else was at the fetes?

PATTY   Oh, clothes ... Jeans![33]

The jean stall proved to be one of the most popular attractions.

The fete drew thousands of people to the Cottages and raised substantial funds. As it was always held on a weekend, securing takings until the bank's opening on the following Monday was essential. Jeannette Hodgkinson, the daughter of the superintendent, Wilfrid Brady, revealed her father's secret hiding place for the stash, 'I remember Dad would have to sleep with all the money raised under his pillow ... We were always pledged to secrecy about the money, always thousands of dollars.'[34]

Residents not only attended the fete, but some contributed to making it a success. When Patrick Reed lived at Kew, he drove children around the grounds on a train that was normally used to transport the laundry and stores. He recollected, 'They used to use it for the fete ... it was a good little toy.'[35] Andrew Ledwidge loved this ride and called it, 'the old Ghost Train'.[36] Another resident, Hubert, escorted small children on the pony ride. These responsibilities were taken very seriously by residents who also relished the opportunity to meet people who came to Kew for this special day. Patrick stated, 'You meet lots of people ... oh it was good.'[37]

Although Patrick was officially rostered to run the Ghost Train, other residents volunteered their services, sometimes unknowingly to fete organisers. Jack Cotter, recalled one incident in the 1970s which brought amusement to many:

> One year the parents came to me and said: 'Did you think we could open a second gate further down Princess Street?' I said: 'Oh, I dunno about that.' They said: 'If we can get all the necessary permission would you mind?' I said: 'Oh I wouldn't mind.' So they went to the council and they went to the police, and the upshot was they were told that they could open it but they could *only* use it as an exit ... Not as an entrance, not as both, the idea was to bring the traffic in the main gate and out that one. They were going to stop all these traffic snarls that they had at previous fetes. Everything worked all right for a while until [a resident], Seitze, set himself up and started directing cars inside the park, and everybody obeyed him immediately. He was standing there stopping this traffic, and

the next thing the traffic's absolutely ground to a halt, there are car horns tooting and people are so confused, and here he is just standing there with this beatific smile on his face still stopping them … everybody was doing exactly what he told them, and it was absolute chaos! [laughing][38]

The intermingling of residents with the general community at the fetes helped to overcome some of the preconceived ideas, and perhaps even fear, that prevailed about people with intellectual disability. The fete was a festive occasion that appeared to be enjoyed by all. In 2001, with resident numbers dwindling and high fees for public liability insurance, the fete ceased. Thus ended one of the residents' most anticipated events at Kew!

Regular celebrations at the Cottages included Easter and Christmas. These occasions were enjoyed by many residents, staff and some families. Decorations were sometimes hung in the wards, plays were performed, and music rang out from various buildings. In the 1920s and '30s, Ted Rowe recalled that Christmas plays were hosted in the Dining Hall, 'at Christmas time they put on a little show … the staff and the kids … They cleared out the tables and everybody would come and see it … [even] parents came to see it.'[39] Ted did not receive any gifts at Christmas, although he did note that younger children were sometimes given toys, 'At Christmas we never even got any toys. Only the little small kids got them, we didn't get anything.'[40]

Special holidays were popular times for families to visit their relatives. It was bittersweet for residents such as Ted who did not have familial contact:

TED   Yes a lot of them came and visited, oh yes. The parents come and see 'em.

CORINNE   Did you become friendly with anyone?

TED   No, never got friendly with anyone. One of the nurses said to me 'I'll be your parents before the others come'. I was sitting on my own, no parents. It was all right … I just had to put up with it, without them. And when I'd see the others I'd

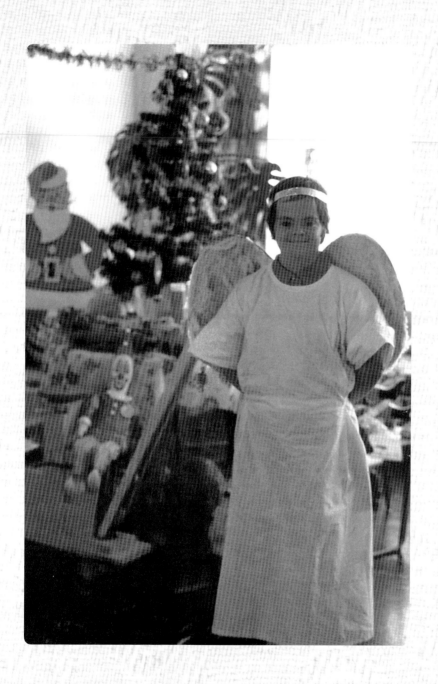

Christmas at Kew Cottages,
circa 1960s. (Courtesy of Kew Cottages
Historical Society)

start to cry and 'Wish I had my mummy and daddy coming to see me.'[41]

Ted was not alone as many residents found themselves in a similar situation.

For a few residents, such as Donald Starick, Easter and Christmas signalled an important time in their lives, moments when they left Kew to spend time with their families:

CORINNE So when you lived at Kew you used to go away for holidays, didn't you?

DONALD Yes. Mum, at Rushworth.

CORINNE And did you enjoy that?

DONALD Yes.

CORINNE And do you still go there?

DONALD Yes.

CORINNE When are you going next? Are you going soon?

DONALD Yes. I'm going, Easter.

CORINNE What's coming up now, what's coming up *this* month?

DONALD Jingle bells.

CORINNE Jingle bells?

DONALD Go home, Christmas.[42]

Unlike Donald, the majority of residents who lived at Kew remained onsite for Easter and Christmas.

Some staff, parents, volunteers and community organisations endeavoured to make Christmas and Easter festive occasions. John Foster was a member of a youth group from the Summerhill Road Methodist Church. He and his associates regularly went to Kew to socialise with residents. John explained that at Christmas time his group made an extra effort, 'When Christmas came around we all drove out there and picked up these young men in Ward 3A and took them back to the church hall and had a Christmas party ... We would buy presents ... mainly food items and cigarettes, what you might call a "Red Cross" parcel.'[43]

Parties were also held onsite and families were invited to come along. As a child, Christine Walton attended Christmas parties that were held in her brother's ward in the 1960s and '70s:

> we always went to the Christmas parties ... They never really felt Christmassy. I always felt that there were lots of people just sitting in the little groups. Mum would talk to the other parents but as a kid I don't remember feeling anything more than this was *not* how a Christmas party should be.[44]

Genuine efforts were made by many people to offer residents enjoyable Christmas and Easter celebrations. Many residents welcomed festivities. In 2006, I visited a community residential unit in which five former Kew residents lived. When Christmas carols were played the men rushed to the living room and sang or hummed along to each song. All of these men had lived at Kew since they were young children. Most had spent Christmas within the institution. This was their first Christmas living in a community residential unit. By the excitement and enthusiasm that filled the living room, for these residents the Christmas celebrations at Kew had created some happy memories.

Kew Cottages often received donations from individuals and groups. These tended to be small, but significant, contributions that offered residents temporary benefits. For example, during World War II the local primary school regularly supplied boxes of fruit to children at the Special School.[45] Individual families some-times made specific donations to remedy poor living conditions in the wards. Geoffrey and Elsie Welchman were unhappy about the freezing conditions in Ward 16A where their son was housed. Being members of the Parents' Association, they were aware of the diffi-culties in obtaining resources for the Cottages and decided to pur-chase heating for the ward. Geoffrey stated, '[there were] no heaters in the unit at all. We provided the strip heaters for him and wherever they needed to warm the hut.[46] The WP O'Shea Research Unit was constructed through a generous donation by another family whose son was a resident at Kew. Initially, this facility provided onsite psycho-therapeutic services and it was later transformed into a community residential unit that offered independent-style accommodation. However, it was two major public appeals, Tipping (1953) and Minus Children (1975), which resulted in substantial improvements in the quality of life for residents at the Cottages.

On 6 April 1953, *Herald* journalist, Bill Tipping, reported that the parents of a six-year-old boy, known as Michael, preferred to tie him to a stake in the backyard than send him to live at 'those terrible Kew Cottages'.[47] Michael was restrained in an effort to maintain his safety. His sister, Mary Scully, recalled, 'my parents had a business, and they were finding it very hard to cope with my brother … he was hyperactive and unfortunately, my parents at times had to tie him to a stake just to keep him from wandering into the street … He was an "escape artist".'[48] A neighbour reported Michael's parents to the police for cruelty. Instead of demonising the parents, Bill Tipping was sympathetic. He personally understood the plight of parents who cared for a child with intellectual disability at home. Officials from the Mental Hygiene Authority met with Michael's parents and encouraged them to place him at Kew. His parents agreed and Michael was admitted to a newly modernised 'Ward F4'. This ward was intended to be a model for the future care of all residents at Kew. Bill Tipping referred to it as an exemplar in his newspaper articles and sought financial support for similar renovations at Kew.

Bill used his journalistic talents to write articles that painted Kew Cottages as a place of hope and despair. He described the poor condition of both the residents and facilities at the institution. Bill observed that a group of children, aged between four to eight years, were enclosed in an asphalted yard, bare footed, groaning and muttering; he called them 'the forgotten people of Kew'.[49] This portrayal starkly contrasted with the upbeat description of the conditions that Michael encountered on his admission. Bill reported that initially Michael had problems settling, but was soon happy in his new surrounds, making friends with fellow residents. Michael was portrayed as one of the rare privileged residents because he was housed in a modernised unit.

Bill appealed to the Victorian Government to provide £30 000 to modernise all of the wards at Kew. The reaction to his plea was an avalanche of letters of support and donations of money, goods and services from the general public. Within days of his first article on Michael, the Tipping Appeal was officially launched with the full support of the *Herald* and radio station 3DB. Tipping challenged the Government to match pound for pound money that was raised via public subscription. The Government agreed and had to match £24 000 donated by members of the public.[50]

Despite the success of the campaign, renovations were slow. Eighteen months after the Appeal very little had been done. Government 'red-tape' was blamed for delays. Victorian premier, John Cain, explained that the public service system was primarily at fault, but also indicated that workmen refused to stay onsite because of 'nauseating' working conditions.[51] It took several years before most improvements were made. By 1960, over 250 additional residents were admitted to the Cottages. Inadequate government resources to meet this increased demand meant that facilities once again fell into disrepair. For Michael, the benefits of being at the centre of the Tipping Appeal were short-lived. Two years after his admission to Kew he was transferred to one of the worst accommodation areas at the Cottages, 'Little Pell'.

In 1975, another public appeal was launched to provide a higher standard of living for residents at the Cottages. This fundraising effort was spearheaded by Kew's coordinator of volunteers, Val Smorgon and was known as the Minus Children Appeal. Val was frustrated by the lack of facilities for residents at Kew. With the support of her close friend, Lillian Frank and other influential allies, she launched a campaign to raise money to build a new kindergarten. She recalled:

We were wanting to build a kindergarten where our volunteers could take the children. I went and had a look at a lot of the Kew Kindergartens and I thought, '$150 000 would be plenty', which in those days it was a lot of money, and 'How am I going to raise $150 000?' So, with Lillian's help, we decided we would run a campaign for $150 000, it ended up being a million.[52]

Val and Lillian approached Victoria's premier, Rupert Hamer, for Government support and he agreed to match public donations dollar for dollar. Val recollected, 'He didn't know we were going to raise a million, so he had to give us a million! ... But he was wonderful and *The Age* newspaper was also very involved, without them we couldn't have done it.'[53]

The media were crucial in stimulating public donations while raising awareness about the degraded nature of State care for people with intellectual disability. Articles printed in *The Age* used emotive images and language to describe the challenges faced by residents living at the Cottages. *The Age* reporter, John Larkin, stated, 'We called them The Minus Children, not to downgrade them, not to imply they were lesser beings, but because they were behind, in everything from esteem to opportunity.'[54] However, sometimes reportage did in fact dehumanise residents. This was evident in an article published in 1975 which used a variety of impersonal ways to describe residents, including the following passage, 'Today the dolls, these clockwork children out of their minds and out of their bodies – for to be retarded can mean you have everything wrong – are blessed with soft sunshine.'[55]

The Minus Children Appeal significantly contributed to the transformation of life at Kew Cottages. The money raised was used to build facilities that served as important centres for education, training, therapy and recreation. However, it took a few years before problems associated with centre staffing and adequate program delivery were resolved. Many residents, such as Ralph Dawson, enjoyed spending time in the Minus Children's buildings. He stated, 'I used to work with all the art staff in Perkins ... it's closed now ... I miss all the art staff.'[56] The Perkin building was named after the editor for *The Age*, Graham Perkin, whose support was vital in ensuring the success of the campaign. His contribution was acknowledged by Rupert Hamer, 'Graham had the right mixture of aggression, humility and editorial brilliance to make the whole idea exciting to the public.'[57] Even though public interest in Kew Cottages waned as the Appeal wound down, the subject of Victoria's treatment of people with disabilities was firmly placed on the public and political agenda. Nine years after the Appeal, Victoria introduced major legislation, the *Intellectually Disabled Persons' Services Act* 1986. Many of the injustices highlighted by the Minus Children Appeal were addressed in the new legislation.

The history of Kew Cottages was predominantly one of inadequacies and problems associated with running a large institution. However, within this often deprived and harsh world were people who exhibited concern and kindness towards residents. Although some peoples' benevolence and interest were short-lived and sometimes even conditional, it nonetheless resulted in positive outcomes for many Kew residents.

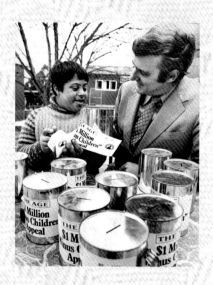

Victorian Health Minister Mr Scanlon, raising
money for the Minus Children Appeal, 1975.
(Courtesy of *The Age* Archives/
The Age, Melbourne)

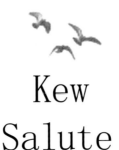

CHAPTER 9

Kew
Salute

*Residents who were scared ... when approached
they cower and cover up and put their hands
up, that was known around the place as a 'Kew
Salute' ... You would get that now, just by
walking past certain people, whether they know
you or not ... It's nothing to be proud of and
it's not a good thing. You probably find a lot of
people wouldn't want to speak about it, but I'll
guarantee every single one of them would know
what you're talking about when you say it.*
Michael Glenister, Kew staff, 15 November 2005

The creation of euphemistic terms such as 'Kew Salute', 'Thump
Therapy' and 'Midnight Special' reflected a violent subculture that
existed at Kew. The use of physical force by some institutional staff
was accepted as necessary to control some residents. However, Kew
Cottages was not a place of punishment for offenders, but a facility
that offered specialised care for one of society's most disadvantaged
groups of people. Many parents who placed their children at Kew
were under the impression that although physical living conditions
were often Spartan, the institution itself was a safe and secure
environment. In reality, Kew Cottages has a confronting history of

violence and abuse which has involved staff, residents, visitors and outsiders at varying times. Unfortunately, as with many institutions, it was not a 'safe haven' but rather a dog-eat-dog world where physical and psychological violence and abuse were ever-present.

The use of aggressive control mechanisms by staff was often justified as essential to maintain order within the institution. Originally, each Cottage was intended to house 20 people, but within a matter of years the demand for places far exceeded availability. The staff-to-resident ratio varied over time, but it was not unusual for one staff member to be responsible for up to 40 residents, during the day, and could be as high as one staff for 80 to 100 residents at night. As life was strictly scheduled, many staff used physical 'encouragement' to hasten daily tasks. One example of this approach was the 'clip over the ear' at mealtimes to force residents to eat quickly.[1] At other times violence was used to exert power and to punish.

Predominantly, victims of staff violence and abuse tended to be ambulant, male residents who were above eight years of age. When I raised the subject of violence with staff members, those who were willing to address the issue often indicated that there was a general understanding that mistreatment of residents with high and complex support needs was taboo. Residents with challenging behaviours were particularly problematic for staff. Kew employee, Michael Glenister, recalled that with the 'more aggressive and violent sorts of residents, there'd be more violence and aggression used by staff associated with them'.[2] Not only did this group of residents threaten the safety of staff, residents and sometimes themselves, many also purposefully undermined institutional regulations.

Periodically, staff were required to use physical force and restraint for protection purposes. According to nurse, Julie Carpenter, some of the residents were very disturbed and exhibited violent behaviours including biting, scratching, punching and serious physical assault.[3] Former chief executive officer (CEO), Max Jackson, supported Julie's account and described the behaviour of an infamous female resident, 'there was a woman there ... you could be standing talking to her and she would then whip out her fingers and poke people in the eye, and that'd be done instantaneously'.[4] Programs were specially devised for many of these residents in order to modify harmful behaviours. For example, the female resident mentioned above was issued with boxing gloves to restrict her movements. Although this approach appears primitive in 2007, it was an acceptable form of restraint in institutions until the 1980s.

Physical and chemical restraints were often used in mental health institutions throughout Western societies to suppress residents' violent behaviours. Staff at Kew were often required to seek official consent before employing restraint. John Wakefield recalled that a powerful chemical regime was commonly used to control male residents in his wards and that aggressive men were routinely given Sodium Amytal.[5] Julie Carpenter described various physical restraint methods that were exercised:

JULIE   There was a lot of physical restraint in those days.

CORINNE   Was that something that was sanctioned by the management at the time?

JULIE   Yes. Basically, they'd say: 'Put it down on paper that you needed to do that.' That was the restraint order. Sometimes it was to prevent them damaging themselves.

CORINNE   What other types of physical restraints were available to staff?

JULIE   Sometimes it would be wrist restraints, they might have their arms tied to the side of a chair, sometimes their legs were tied as well, sometimes it would be a big padded helmet, so they couldn't bash on walls, sometimes it might be a whole harness, a netting harness that was tied to the chair. Boxing gloves to stop them injuring themselves or scratching other people.[6]

Permission was sought in some cases, but at other times staff unofficially utilised makeshift restraints, such as straightjackets made from cloth nappies or gowns.

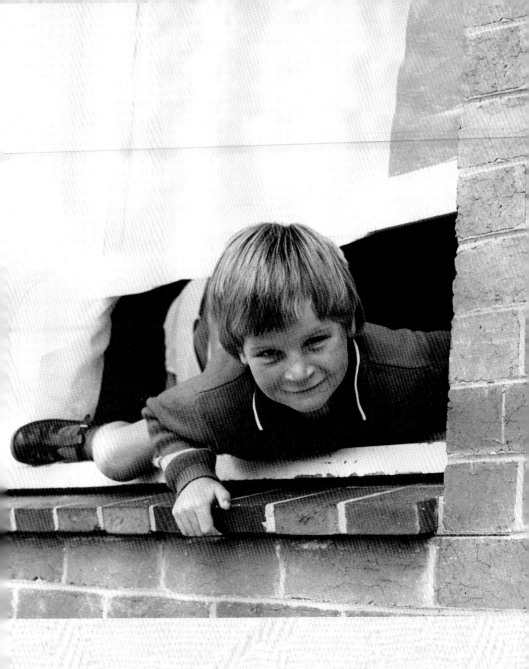

A resident 'escaping' the confines of his ward, Minus Children Appeal, 1975. (Courtesy of *The Age* Archives/*The Age*, Melbourne)

Although physical force was exerted by staff for protection purposes, it was also used as punishment for challenging staff, absconding, failing to obey orders and creating trouble. Popular methods of punishing residents included the cane, strap, slap or 'clip over the ear'. Resident Patrick Reed was sometimes physically reprimanded for 'bad behaviour':

PATRICK They used to hit you with the strap, you know they had a strap. And they're like leather, like the Nuns used to have.

CORINNE And this was at Kew?

PATRICK Yes.

CORINNE And they'd hit you with the strap?

PATRICK Mm [nodding].

CORINNE Where would they hit you?

PATRICK On the hand. If you pull your hand away you get another one.[7]

Until the late 20th century, these punishments were standard practice, not only in other institutions, but also in many schools and family homes throughout Australia.[8] In fact, corporal punishment in Victorian schools was only outlawed in 1983. Kew's regulations strictly forbade the use of physical force in this manner. Staff who utilised these methods were in direct contravention of established mental health guidelines.

The often secretive nature of violence and abuse at the Cottages meant that such activities were rarely officially reported with a code of silence governing working life within the wards. Social worker, Fran van Brummelen, recalled that 'A lot of abuse was covered up by nursing staff because you don't squeal on your peers.'[9] If a staff member was suspected of inappropriate behaviour, then those who worked closely with him/her preferred to address the situation and dole out reprimands. This was a typical form of institutional reaction and resulted in an inaccurate record of the level of violence being perpetrated at the Cottages. In addition, some staff considered violence to be a manifest part of institutional life. Michael Glenister stated:

> I think you need to pretty much accept that in a lot of respects institutions are brutal places. You can watch the movies on TV about prisoners and there's a top dog and then there's a hierarchy and all that sort of stuff. That's the same in any institution, and there's I suppose there's top dogs when it comes to the staff ... to say that you never saw any staff being heavy-handed or whatever, you'd be naïve to say that, that nothing like that ever went on.[10]

Whistleblowers risked being ostracised by colleagues if they lodged official complaints. Some community visitors witnessed the bullying and intimidation of staff who were perceived to be working against the status quo. One community visitor was adamant that, 'if the staff are bullying each other, they'd be bullying the residents'.[11]

When he was CEO, Max Jackson knew that some staff participated in violent activities at Kew, but found it difficult to obtain substantive evidence. Max noted that offending 'staff are pretty cunning in terms of when and how they would do things'.[12] On occasion, when complaints of staff violence were filed with management, action was taken according to the severity of the act. Kurt Kraushofer stated that when he was assistant head nurse, on receipt of a report of suspected violence and abuse, he:

> intervened immediately. It wasn't allowed. When something like this happened in an institution like Kew you couldn't hide it because there was always another staff member around or another client who could talk ... When it happened actions were taken and we called the police in when it was appropriate, and when it was not appropriate we managed it ourselves.[13]

John Wakefield was perturbed at not being able to prove abuse by suspected staff members, 'if I could have proved it I would have! There are some people that you're not quite sure about, but you've got to get the evidence, and most times you can't'.[14]

In the 1970s, Kew's superintendent, Gary McBrearty, established 'bruise books' to record resident injuries and to undertake investigations that he considered to be necessary. These manuals were commonly used in institutional settings as a means of ensuring that attention was drawn to physical injury and its prevention, while also making staff accountable for the welfare of residents. The books were placed in each ward at Kew and were regularly collected and inspected by the superintendent. Manager, Jack Cotter noted that Gary was fastidious in reading these books.[15] He was obviously concerned with eliminating abusive behaviour at the Cottages. However, despite these accountability measures, violence and abuse continued.

On occasion, residents complained about staff violence. Some even used the hierarchical institutional system to ensure that their discontent reached top management. This was certainly evident when the superintendent's son, Philip Brady, was asked to intervene on behalf of a disgruntled resident, Patrick Reed. Patrick was hit several times by a male staff member when he questioned an umpiring decision at a recreational cricket game in his ward. Upset by the attack, Patrick saw Philip walking through the grounds and took the opportunity to seek his help. He asked Philip to tell his father about the incident telling him, 'the staff were hitting me'.[16] On hearing Patrick's version of events, Philip apparently replied, '"I'll get my Dad to go straight down there".'[17] Wilfrid Brady responded to the complaint by speaking with Patrick about the incident and duly reprimanded the staff member in question.[18] Being the superintendent's son carried privilege, a status that was clearly recognised and sometimes utilised by residents at the institution. Patrick recalled that after that episode the staff member in question never hit him again, 'he used to hit me, but then he stopped'.[19]

Many residents who were victims of staff violence understood that there was a reward and punishment system that operated at Kew. If residents 'behaved' and followed orders they were relatively safe from punishment. Resident, Ted Rowe, recalled what it was like in the 1920s and '30s:

TED We never had any slapping or anything. Some did, they'd annoy the nurse and they'd say 'Get the cane' and whack you ... And gee they hurt too.

CORINNE If you did something wrong you'd get the cane?

TED Yeah, I had it a couple of times.

CORINNE What for? What did you do?

TED Said something I shouldn't have said.[20]

Ted believed that residents had to take some responsibility for their actions, 'Someone said they treated us like dogs. Well I said "it was your fault, I haven't been treated like a dog". I just did what I was told, see, that was it ... I didn't get in much trouble ... I behaved myself.'[21]

Although female residents suffered from staff violence and abuse, its prevalence appeared to be far less than their male counterparts. A reason for this disparity may have been due to the fact that up until the 1960s, the male division was run by men who adhered to contemporary ideals of masculinity based upon physicality. Historian, Henry Reynolds, argued that masculinity in Australia was often measured by a man's ability to fight, '"Real men" were expected to be tough, to be handy with their fists and ever ready for a fight. Their women were frequently subject to their aggression as were "poofters" or "dagos" or anyone else who looked different.'[22] Male residents were often treated roughly by staff, sometimes as punishment, other times in the belief that they were toughening them up to become 'real men'. These behaviours were learned by many male residents who then brutalised those residents less powerful than themselves.

Prior to the 1960s, many male staff appeared to show little compassion for residents and frequently used aggressive physical and psychological methods to manage their charges. One reason for the introduction of female staff into male wards was to curb this type of behaviour. Staff member, John Wakefield, was pleased with this institutional change:

Medical Violence

Violence was not always an intentional act of
punishment and control. At times it was an
inherent part of the world in which people
lived. The following story highlights the cruel
reality of life at Kew Cottages for residents
who received medical treatment without the
benefits of pain relief:

There was one chap, he was about 6 foot 3 inches
and he was stooped. The airing court gate that
time had these pointed wood pickets, and he
used to leap it ... he must have misstepped and
as he did, he tore his scrotum and a testicle
fell down. Nobody saw this happen, but that is
what happened, and we found him in a pool of
blood. So, we took him down to the ward and
then phoned Dr Cantor, a man with a sense of
humour. He came down to the ward and, in those
days, there was no anaesthetic issued, you just
held them as sutures were being inserted. He got
the testicle in, made three more sutures, applied
acriflavine, and I said, 'now will there be any
further treatment, doctor?' He said, 'postpone his
honeymoon for another 3 weeks'.

(Interview between Cliff Judge and Ted Wilson, Kew Cottages
Historical Society, circa 1987)

[It] just changed the whole attitude, particularly the male attitudes.
I know I had a couple of very remarkable ladies ... who came in and
softened up the unit. They were the 'mothers'. They were usually
older women with experience with their own kids ... They took away
that blokey military approach.[23]

Fran van Brummelen supported John's claims, 'Just having female
staff in a male unit changed the climate completely ... there'd be

much less aggressive behaviour.'[24] However, some female staff were not averse to using physical violence to control their wards. As Clare Turner testified, during the 1960s and '70s she was struck by female staff members for refusing to eat her porridge.[25] Gradually, the use of violence changed as social attitudes towards its acceptability also altered. From the 1970s more conciliatory approaches to behaviour management were introduced to deal with staff-resident relations and challenging behaviours.

Aggressive physical management had a lasting impact on many residents. Michael Glenister testified to the continued power of male staff in the 21st century:

> I can walk into a room and I can raise my voice now and people say: 'Gee, how did you get such control over them?' And it's purely because I'm male. And it's purely because, for whatever reason over time, residents have not revered males, but been maybe scared of them or more inclined to do what they're told and I've benefited from that.[26]

Psychological abuse was also apparent at the Cottages. Julie Carpenter revealed that some staff were prone to use:

> mental torture, perhaps teasing them, withholding things that were very important to them, because not many of them had individual possessions and if they did have something little that they wanted to hold onto, then staff could see by taking it away, that was a way of punishing them.[27]

Max Jackson believed that some staff were abusive in order to gain a sense of power, 'there were certainly a number of staff who I think psychologically abused clients, but I think any environment, any human service environment attracts people who have their own needs, that is their own need to be in charge, their own need to be noticed'.[28] Max collaborated with senior staff members and union officials to try and overhaul this practice. Although strategic plans were made at a management level, enforcing these strategies in the units was a major hurdle. Psychological abuse was a long-term problem that persisted even beyond Max's reforms. This type of control mechanism was common, particularly when physical punishment was no longer tolerated.

On occasion a few staff members engineered situations which resulted in violent altercations or abusive behaviours by residents. Max Jackson recalled, 'It wasn't uncommon for staff, almost as a sport, to goad a client against another client.'[29] Although some people likened this behaviour to the type of antics that many apprentices endured in the mainstream community, this was an intentional misuse of staff power that sometimes resulted in injury and harm. Kew staff member, Jan Sharp, was the victim of what was meant to be a prank:

> The staff ... used to teach some of the boys rather nasty sexual habits, and one of them was a young lad ... in his 20s ... they taught him ... that when he saw a woman coming towards him in a skirt he had to say: 'I'd like to f[uck] you' and promptly put his hand up your skirt ... Anyway, I'll probably get myself into trouble, but I hit him. I hit him really hard because, number one, *nobody* does that to me, I don't like being touched at the best of times, least of all being told that and a hand rammed up your skirt. I mean it was so quick that I got taken unawares, and I hit him. I grabbed hold of him by the arms and I said: 'If you *ever* do that again ... I'll hurt you so *badly* you won't know what's happened to you.' He never came near me after that.[30]

In 2006, Jan laughingly recounted this story with sympathy for the resident who was set up by conniving staff. However, at the time, she was furious. Doubtless the resident was also traumatised by being so severely reprimanded. What was considered to be fun and games for a few staff caused physical pain and humiliation for the resident and Jan.

Although some staff were intentionally violent, on occasion others failed to recognise the harmful nature of their actions when denying residents basic care. This was certainly the case when Helen Wilson witnessed a colleague failing in his duty of care:

> I remember an instance where I actually saw a staff member throwing a resident's drink down the sink rather than giving it to them, and when they tried to deny that they had done it I said: 'Look I saw you, why did you do that?' It was to make himself look good, that he had done a good job and he was quick and efficient.[31]

Helen explained the possible health implications to the staff member. She stressed the fact that efficient work practices were not necessarily associated with speed, but rather quality of service. She forthrightly declared, 'I think people with that sort of attitude shouldn't *be* here.'[32]

Staff were not the sole perpetrators of violence and abuse at Kew. Resident violence and abuse was a constant problem and was most prevalent in wards where older children and adults were housed together. Until the 1960s, children aged up eight years, were mostly cared for by female staff in the Nursery and children's wards. According to most interviewees, these wards were the most loving, enjoyable and rewarding places to reside and work. When children were transferred out of these wards they were sent to live in dormitories with people of varying ages. Housing was based upon need, rather than age. Inevitably, many younger residents were bullied by their more mature counterparts. John Wakefield stated, 'There was an enormous amount of bastardisation, and bullying by the older boys to the younger boys, they always did it very badly when they moved across … People can sweep it under the carpet and say it didn't happen, but it was very real, and it was a problem.'[33] Resident, Clare Turner, also recounted various times when she was assaulted by people living in her ward. On one occasion:

CLARE   I was on my bed … doing the socks with the night duty lady and one girl come up and bit me on the nose right on my skin the whole lot.

CORINNE   What happened?

CLARE   And then I, I was crying.

CORINNE   Did anyone help you?

CLARE   Well the lady saw me there: 'What's wrong', I go: 'Well what's going on?' and then she go: 'Oh, look at *you*' … gee they pushed me around so much in that place.[34]

Clare also broke her arm when residents intentionally pushed her out of her wheelchair. On weekends when her parents brought her home, Clare dreaded Sunday afternoons. She was upset about leaving her parents and feared what lay before her at Kew, 'I started crying, I couldn't take it.'[35]

One of the common forms of resident violence was the 'Midnight Special'. When I asked residents Ralph Dawson and Andrew Ledwidge what this meant they replied:

RALPH A snoogle, a snoogle-snuckles in his head, one of these ones [gesturing by raising a fist to his head, indicating a punch] up on his head.

CORINNE What's a snoogle-snuckle?

RALPH Andrew Ledwidge will know what it is, he will understand.

ANDREW Snoogles are 'Midnight Special'.

CORINNE And who would get a Midnight Special?

ANDREW A Midnight Special?

CORINNE Why would somebody get a Midnight Special, what would they do to warrant getting a Midnight Special?

RALPH Annoy people.

CORINNE And did you ever get one?

RALPH No, I'm clever, that's why isn't it Andy Ledwidge?

ANDREW Yes.[36]

Over the weeks that followed our interview, whenever I tried to elicit information about who taught them about the 'Midnight Special', Ralph and Andrew avoided the subject. This was a fascinating example of the extension of institutional silence carried into the community; I was allowed to know that the act had occurred, but not who the specific teachers or perpetrators were.

Sexual abuse was a major concern at the Cottages. This was one reason why the gender division was initially established. Kurt and Maria Kraushofer worked in a variety of wards at Kew from the 1950s. They stated that abusive behaviour was most prevalent among male residents who they considered to be more sexually active than their female counterparts.[37] Fran van Brummelen shared this viewpoint and when asked about this subject replied, that there was:

> sexual abuse between *residents*, a lot of homosexual incidents. I mean what do you expect? Dormitories with say 20 teenagers, locked at night, because there was only one person on at night, and there were two dormitories. There might be 48 people with one person, and of course there were episodes.[38]

Staff members, such as Michael Glenister and John Wakefield, were aware of bastardisation that occurred in the male units and tried to teach residents behaviour modification, or provide protection for potential victims. Michael noted:

> I used to feel sorry for some of the residents. During the day there was plenty of staff around, they'd be protected, but in some of the male units there was a whole lot of inappropriate sexual activity that went on … if there were staff around who could protect them that is all well and good, but some of the residents were quite cunning and manipulating, and brutalised other residents when the staff weren't around.[39]

The role of staff in preventing resident abuse was critical, but as understaffing was a constant problem, many residents were exposed to violent exploitation.

Sexual abuse of female residents was also a concern at the institution, but did not appear to be as rampant as among the male population. Up until the 1960s, gender segregation was designed to prohibit sexual contact between male and female residents. Although a few people circumvented this division when possible, relationships and pregnancies appeared to be rare. When male and female residents began to live in mixed units from the 1960s, human relations classes were introduced to teach them about consent issues and sexual rights. These lessons were meant to ensure that sexual abuse was avoided. However, occasionally violence and abuse occurred. Melanie Shield was the victim of a rape perpetrated by a male resident in her unit. This information came to the fore after she told her sister Emily of the attack. No action was taken against the alleged attacker because of a lack of evidence. After this incident, when Melanie's family came to Kew, they were continually confronted by the alleged rapist who mocked them with verbal abuse and obscene gestures.[40]

Staff were also wary of being accused of sexual abuse. This concern was noted by Kurt and Maria Kraushofer who spoke candidly about the issue:

KURT Can I also come back to an interesting part and that's about sexuality. Maria worked in the Princess Street houses with people of 40, 50 years of age and the big thing in the mid-90s was sexuality and family planning. It even got to the extent that they bought hundreds of penises and vaginas and showed how to use them to people in Kew. There was one lady who came to the houses and told Maria that she should show people how to put a condom on. You tell your story now.

MARIA Yeah and I just said: 'Are you mad?' I said: 'And he's going to go all around Kew saying: "Maria touched my penis."' She said 'Okay, maybe you can ask Kurt to show him?' Anyway I came home and said to him 'Would you put the condom on Richard?' And he said 'Are you mad, so he can go and say I touched him?'

KURT I play with his doodle.

MARIA So I went back and I said to Kathy: 'Actually you're a family planner, it's your job, why don't you touch his penis?'

CORINNE What was her response?

MARIA 'I don't think that is appropriate.'[41]

Kurt and Maria were aware of the dangers of false accusation as they had witnessed other people, whom they considered to be innocent, accused of inappropriate behaviour. They cited one incident:

KURT [There] was a very outgoing young girl. We had a volunteer who used to be a firefighter. When people used to come in she always came running and gave them a hug. Some freedom fighter seen that and reported it.

MARIA And he was investigated.

KURT We had to tell that poor man …

MARIA Not to come near.

KURT 'Don't come near!' Basically accusing him, it was very sad.

MARIA It was awful.[42]

Anecdotal evidence suggests that a few staff were involved in inappropriate sexual behaviour with residents. However due to the clandestine nature of these activities, the extent to which it occurred at Kew will never be known.

Families were sometimes aware of violence being perpetrated against their relatives and were even victims of violence. Rosalie Trower's son, Stephen, was admitted to Kew in 1982. On weekends, Rosalie often took Stephen home. She was perturbed by bruises and scratches that were all over Stephen's body. She discovered that he was being regularly attacked by a fellow resident in his unit. One Monday around lunchtime, Rosalie returned Stephen to the Cottages after a home visit. She parked her car near Stephen's unit and was about to open her car door when they were seized upon:

> there was a fellow … who was set to kill Steve … this fellow appeared, out of the blue, made a dive at Steve's side, I banged the buttons down so he couldn't open the doors, he then threw himself on the bonnet, shouted and screamed, there was *nobody* around because they were at lunch … As I locked the doors, I thought: 'There's only one way out of this, just drive out, get out of the place', so I did.[43]

Rosalie drove to the Administration building and met with Max Jackson and Fran van Brummelen. She demanded that Stephen be immediately moved to another unit. The only available alternative was a unit that was terribly overcrowded, but Rosalie agreed to the transfer in order to protect her son. She was angry that she had to resolve the situation, 'he was safe there, of course, [but] *I had* to do that'.[44] Stephen was fortunate that his mother recognised the abuse and demanded action. Many other residents endured continual abuse as they had little or no family contact or advocates who were willing or able to assist.

The violent and criminal behaviours of some residents were sometimes so severe that they were sent to alternate mental health and violent offenders' institutions. This was certainly the case in the 1940s, when a male resident attempted to drown another man at the Cottages. This offender was considered to be too dangerous for the Cottages and was transferred to Kew Mental Hospital. Shortly afterwards he killed a fellow resident by hitting him over the head with a broom.[45]

Young residents were also involved in violent episodes at Kew. Jack and Margaret Cotter recalled that in the 1970s, when they worked at Kew, there was a pair of boys who were considered by staff to be extremely dangerous and who terrorised residents at the institution. At the age of nine they stole puppies from the local guide dog facility, which were never seen again. They often absconded and perpetrated criminal offences. Jack and Margaret recollected:

JACK I think he was a junior psychopath actually, because he was positively dangerous, yet he was angelic looking. I can remember the nursing staff saying the day they came to take him to Baltara … The people who came and took him were looking at the staff as much to say …

MARGARET 'You mean lot!'

JACK Yes. 'You mean lot, sending this dear little boy away' … They were no sooner out there than they broke into every house in the whole area.

CORINNE What happened in those situations, were the police called in to deal with any of these events?

MARGARET Not really. They finished up, well he was only about 12 when he went up to J Ward ... Then he was in Pentridge.[46]

A few residents exhibited extreme violence. These people were often dealt with through relocation or physical and chemical restraint. In later years behavioural management programs were introduced.

Although a lot of violence emanated from people working and residing within the institution, a few visitors and outsiders were also a danger. Kew Cottages was well known as an institution that housed vulnerable people. Unfortunately, facilities such as State homes, schools and hospitals, often attracted predators looking for potential victims. Residents and staff were exposed to criminal acts committed by outside offenders. In the 1970s a nurse was brutally raped in the grounds on her way to the Nurses' Home. The perpetrator was known to have worn a woollen hat. However, as Jack Cotter noted, around 90 per cent of residents at Kew wore woollen hats at this time, so this piece of evidence was not helpful. It was generally believed that the rapist was an outsider.[47]

On another occasion, a young female resident was raped. Emily Shield visited her sister Melanie regularly each Saturday. One day, as Emily was leaving, she dropped Melanie off at the onsite social club which opened regularly on Saturday afternoons. Tragically, on this occasion the club remained shut and Melanie was kidnapped by a stranger. He raped her and sent her back to the Administration building, in a taxi, with a bag of lollies. Even though Emily was in no way responsible, she clearly blamed herself for the assault on her sister, 'I left her there'.[48] The rape was reported to the police and Melanie was interviewed. Emily was furious during police questioning when Melanie was asked, 'Did you enjoy this?'[49] Melanie was a rape victim twice, but neither man was prosecuted.

Many residents were unwilling or incapable of officially reporting incidents of violence and abuse. Some of these people resorted to violent means to unofficially deal with problems. Others, with severe disabilities or communication issues, were unable to effectively lodge a complaint, or were unaware that abuse was even taking place. These vulnerable residents were often reliant upon knowledgeable and sympathetic staff who knew them well to recognise abuse. The community visitors were acutely aware of this difficulty:

> It's always going to be difficult because the person isn't able to [tell you] ... Sometimes we've been told by a day program [service] ... that people won't get off the bus when they come back [to Kew], if there's a certain person at the unit. I've attended a few of the programs with [these] people. I found at a particular unit that I was visiting that several people wouldn't get off the bus, and they were convinced that there was a problem.[50]

Gut feelings and supposition were not enough for official action to be taken by Kew management. Therefore, some dedicated staff and visitors helped residents through direct intervention. In the early 1980s, when employed as a team leader in the Hamer Centre, Alma Adams was certain that abuse was taking place:

> There was one unit here ... when you went in and walked *near* the clients they'd all sort of move away, it was just really, really scary. The atmosphere just felt wrong. I mean many people felt like that, nothing ever came out of it, nobody knew anything, but the whole environment *felt* abusive. This is not a criticism of the people who were *managing* at the time, because there was never any evidence, it was just something that you knew. We tried all sorts of ways to get rid of that by having program staff going in there in the morning, so that you might try and break some of the culture down a little bit, [and by] having more people coming and going ... [so] if anything untoward was going on you'd have a better chance of it actually being seen and coming out ... You can speculate about what was happening and who was responsible, but it's nothing more than speculation because you could never get underneath it all.[51]

Kew staff called upon the police to deal with some allegations of resident violence. This procedure was introduced in the late 20th century and caused discontent among some people, particularly family members who believed that residents were being unnecessarily punished for minor altercations that could have been handled more appropriately in-house. Police were called to Melanie Shield's unit after she pushed a fellow resident. Apparently, this incident caused no physical injury to the parties involved. Melanie and her family were very upset that the duty staff were unable to deal with the episode and instead called in the police. Melanie stated, 'They called the police out to me … I was sad … I don't want them to [come]. It's not right.'[52] This policy may not have been popular among staff if the tables had been turned and residents had been openly encouraged and taught to phone the police when staff exhibited similar behaviours! Although police were involved in some altercations at Kew, despite official policy many staff preferred to resolve conflicts without this type of intervention.

Kew Cottages was a harsh place in which to live. The struggle for superiority in the institutional hierarchy; desperate attempts for attention; constant boredom and a lack of behavioural programs to manage challenging behaviours; all contributed to the violent and abusive behaviours exerted by many staff and residents. However, John Wakefield considered that violence is inherent in some people, 'some people are born bastards'.[53] Despite the determined efforts of some staff, visitors and families to prevent violence and abuse, it was a dark feature of institutional life.

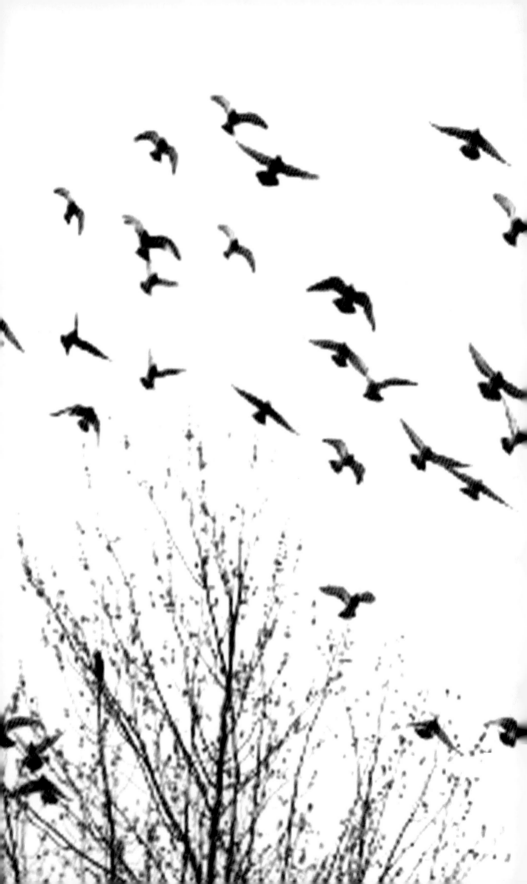

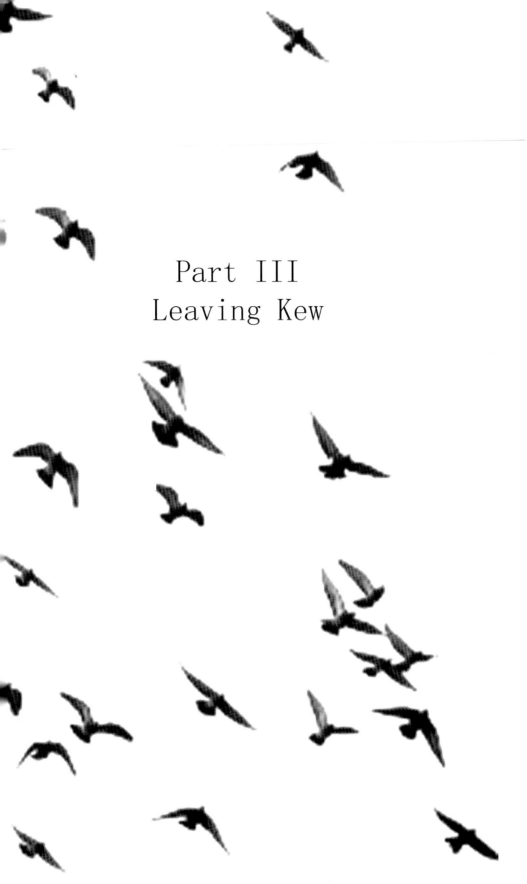

Part III
Leaving Kew

*Miss Lucas got me out, she did, but anyhow,
I wanted to move on because I'd been there
for a long time.*

Lois Philmore, resident, 25 January 2007

Sadly, for many residents, their final journey from Kew was through the onsite mortuary. Some families came to share the last moments of their relatives' lives and claimed their bodies for burial. However, as many residents did not have family contact, their deaths often went unmarked. A major exception to this rule was related to the deaths of nine men in a fire at Kew in 1996. Their passing caused public outcry and their funeral and memorial services drew hundreds of attendees and media attention. The following chapter, 'Walking Ghosts', explores the impact of the fire from the perspective of people most closely associated with the tragedy.

Throughout the years, many residents, such as Lois Philmore, expressed a desire to leave Kew and live in the general community. However, a lack of State funded community care facilities meant most residents remained confined to the institution. From the 1980s, government deinstitutionalisation programs hastened the relocation of residents from State-run institutions into community housing. A small number of Kew residents were re-housed in semi-independent and independent accommodations, such as Moorakyne Hostel. As institutions closed, residents for whom accommodation could not be found in the community were often sent to the Cottages. This was the case for James Barry Woods and Barry Evans who were transferred from Sunbury. The 1996 fire was a catalyst that highlighted the negative implications of large-scale care and contributed to the Victorian Government's decision to close Kew Cottages. The final chapter in this history explores the response of various people to the closure and redevelopment plans for Kew. It reveals that this was a highly contentious and emotive issue.

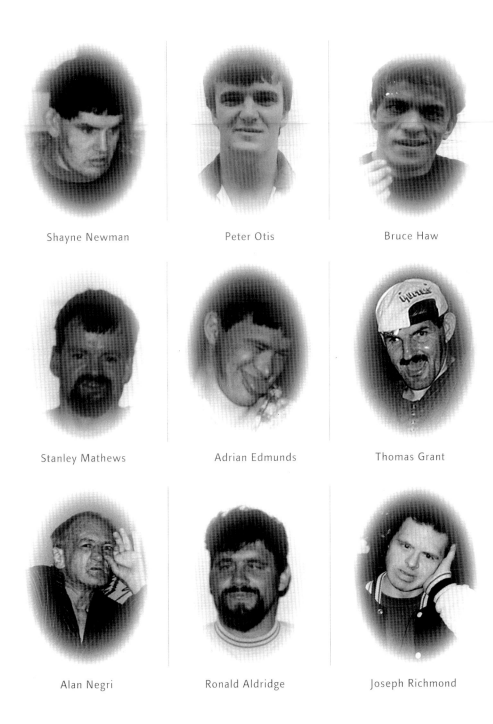

Shayne Newman

Peter Otis

Bruce Haw

Stanley Mathews

Adrian Edmunds

Thomas Grant

Alan Negri

Ronald Aldridge

Joseph Richmond

The nine residents who perished on 8 April 1996. (Courtesy of Kew Residential
Services, Department of Human Services, Victoria)

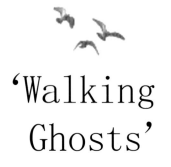

CHAPTER 10

'Walking Ghosts'

RONALD ALDRIDGE
ADRIAN EDMUNDS
THOMAS GRANT
BRUCE HAW
STANLEY MATHEWS
ALAN NEGRI
SHAYNE NEWMAN
PETER OTIS
JOSEPH RICHMOND

One cold, rainy night in April 1996 these nine men, between 31 and 61 years of age, were killed in a fire that swiftly and violently engulfed their unit at Kew Cottages. Throughout its history, over 2000 residents have died at Kew, some in horrifying circumstances. Most of these deaths were single or isolated events that drew little, if any, public attention. By contrast, the 1996 fire sent shockwaves throughout the Australian and international communities. In a State care facility that was meant to look after vulnerable people, how could so many men die in such harrowing circumstances?

The Coronial Inquest into the fire and deaths revealed that

successive Victorian Governments had failed to provide adequate facilities and care at the Cottages. In a watershed moment in Victorian history, the State was blamed as a key contributor to this catastrophic event. The Coronial and fire investigations resulted in a major overhaul of safety standards across State facilities and hastened the deinstitutionalisation of residents away from the Cottages into mainstream Australian society.[1] A detailed account of the fire was outlined in the findings handed down by Victoria's State Coroner.[2] However, mythology still surrounds the deaths of the nine men. Personal stories of those closely connected to the fire help to debunk some of the prevailing myths and reveal the emotional impact and devastation brought about by this tragedy.

Aside from a couple of anecdotes, no interviewees offered much information about each of the men who died. Perhaps this was a by-product of life inside a large institution, where people sometimes get lost among the crowd. Or maybe interviewees did not want to favour one life over another by offering information about particular victims. Despite being at the heart of the tragedy the victims often remained invisible. The magnitude of the fire overshadowed the loss of individuals. The victims were commonly referred to as 'the nine men'.

For decades concerns had been raised by the Metropolitan Fire Brigade (MFB), staff, parents, community visitors, consultants and experts about fire safety at Kew Cottages.[3] Many people recalled the fire that had killed six female residents at Willsmere in 1968, noting that this was a stark warning of the potential dangers when there were inadequate fire safety measures. The MFB was critical of existing fire safety measures and recommended changes in order to drastically raise standards to protect residents. Unfortunately, for the most part, such advice seems to have fallen on deaf ears. Despite the reticence of the Victorian Government to enact recommended improvements, the MFB tried to ensure that its service was appropriate for protecting the interests of those housed within the institution. An MFB officer, Ronald Haines, stated:

The MFB involvement with Kew Cottages goes back many years, not only through fire calls but through assisting the Cottages with fire safety matters as well. Due to the disability of the clients and the age and construction of some of the buildings it was in the back of minds of firefighters that any real emergency at the Cottages would present the Brigade with particular problems. That is why the Brigade had an enhanced response to the Cottages (normal response is two fire appliances, however the Cottages receive three appliances to every call). This enhanced response gives the Brigade additional resources in the initial stages should an emergency occur. This additional response would prove invaluable during the disastrous fire of April 1996.[4]

In the early 1970s, Ronald Haines was a frequent visitor to Kew Cottages, cashing employees' pay cheques on behalf of the State Savings Bank. In 1976 he joined the MFB and worked as a station officer in various places, including the old Kew Fire Station located in Belford Road. Ron recalled that the relationship between the MFB and Kew Cottages was ongoing and amicable:

During the time I was at the Kew Fire Station I attended many fire calls to the Kew Cottages. The calls were mainly false alarms only a few minor fires; thankfully nothing of significance. However, attending calls I became quite familiar with the layout of the Cottages and also got to know many of the staff and clients. We were always met with great enthusiasm by the clients who wanted to shake our hands and waved to us warmly when we departed the scene. The firefighters always took time out after a fire-call to show clients around the fire appliance and to spend time talking to staff and clients.[5]

Ron was the first officer from the MFB to attend the 1996 fire. He arrived within minutes of the first fire appliances. Unlike many previous visits this was not a false alarm; he was confronted by a scene of destruction and despair.

At approximately 10.49 pm on 8 April 1996, a male resident set light to bedding in a room that he shared with Thomas Grant and Shayne Newman. Over the following seven minutes flames steadily grew, creating choking, poisonous smoke. The two night staff who were in charge of 45 residents in what was popularly known as Unit 30/31, were unaware of the dire events that were about to unfold. At

10.56 pm, the MFB responded to an automatic fire alarm. By 11.01 pm three fire appliances were onsite.

By the time firefighters started to battle the blaze it had taken hold with flames erupting 20 metres in the air. Smoke was billowing from the building and an orange glow lit the night sky. Residents were being evacuated by staff who were summoned from nearby units. Chaos reigned as many terrified and confused residents tried to return to their bedrooms in the burning building. Staff and firefighters were sometimes physically challenged by frightened and dazed evacuees.

Michael Giacomi was among the first group of firefighters to tackle the fire. As he and fellow officer Graham Smith entered the premises through Flat C they were met with thick smoke and intense heat. Michael's description of the desperate situation was heartbreaking and illustrated the obvious terror of those trapped inside:

> When I first arrived on scene I heard a whole lot of screaming and stuff. The screams were not like screams that I had heard before in respects to having been to the Kew Cottages. The patients sometimes get really excited when the fire trucks turn up. These were different screams altogether, they appeared to come from the area that we were trying to attack, it was beyond the area that we could access, where the fire was at the time I was there it was all smoke and the screams were coming from behind the smoke. I was unable to get beyond the door at the end of the small corridor and it appeared this was the main area of the fire and the area where the screams came from.[6]

We will never know exactly who was crying out, but it would appear that three of the victims had tried to escape the inferno. The bodies of Shayne Newman and Thomas Grant were found in the living/kitchen area only metres from an exit door, while Ronald Aldridge was discovered in a passageway near a door leading to a communal lounge room. The remaining men lay within the confines of their bedrooms, some lay on the floor, while others were framed within their metal beds. Many people clung to the hope that these men passed away as they slept or were little aware of the grim situation in which they found themselves. The Coroner concluded that all the men died from carbon monoxide poisoning and burns. An MFB report determined that the deceased died within six minutes and 30 seconds from the fire's ignition.[7] As the fire alarm was not raised until seven minutes 45 seconds later we can assume that the cries Michael heard were not from those who died.

At 12.22 am on 9 April the fire was declared to be 'under control'. By this time the site was a hive of activity. The MFB alone had 113 personnel, 21 fire appliances and 23 other Brigade vehicles in attendance.[8] Other emergency personnel were also onsite and the media were gathering. At around 12.30 am Detective Sergeant Peter O'Connor and Detective Senior Constable Graeme Wheeler of the Criminal Investigation Branch arrived at the fire location. As they drove to Kew, Peter was somewhat apprehensive about what lay ahead, 'It was going to be a daunting task … There was a sense of foreboding about it all. It was Kew Cottages, with retarded people, and the fact that there were going to be dead bodies because of a major fire. So we were fairly apprehensive about it all … and heading over there it was fairly quiet in the car.'[9] Uncertainty was soon overcome as they approached the site of the fire. According to Peter, automatic pilot kicked in and they set about controlling the scene, 'it was fairly disorganised … The scene hadn't been contained. If it's a crime or a serious matter like we had there, the scene's got to be contained, the comings and going of people have to be monitored and recorded. For various reasons, that hadn't been done.'[10] Ambulance officer, Tony Armour, supported Peter's claims, 'When I first arrived on the scene it looked like a major disaster with people running everywhere.'[11] Peter was concerned that the disorderliness could potentially lead to a contamination of a possible crime scene. Fortunately this did not occur.

One of the largest groups of onlookers was the media who were quick to respond to news of a major fire at Kew. Journalists and news personnel photographed, filmed and attempted to interview anyone who could help in collating their stories. Peter O'Connor noted that members of the media were everywhere. On entering a room where residents lost their lives Peter was angered by the presence of media peering into the crime scene:

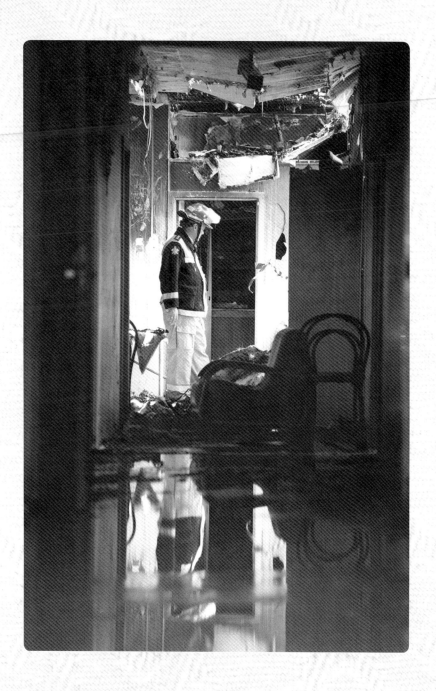

A firefighter standing in Unit 31.
(Courtesy of *Herald and Weekly Times*
Photographic Collection)

> There was a heap of damage to the structure, it was pretty severe.
> From memory there were walls missing … I was in the building and
> I was looking up, and I can see all the cameramen there, it was crazy
> … I have a memory of looking through this hole and seeing the
> media there, and thinking: 'What have they got their noses in here
> for? Get out of here.'[12]

The intrusive nature of media was vividly recorded by news footage
shot that evening. A televised film clip showed a camera crew being
ordered out of the destroyed unit by irate firefighters who were
attempting to bring the situation under control. The media were
driven back to an area away from the immediate fire location.

Despite the growing number of people amassing at Unit 30/31
the atmosphere was solemn, 'It was pretty eerie and dark, and it
was quiet.'[13] With the assistance of fellow police officers, Peter and
Graeme swiftly set about organising a perimeter to stop unauthorised entry by media, staff, residents and members of the general
public. They liaised with the MFB, police forensic investigators and
Kew staff to ascertain the sequence of events. They were informed
that a staff member had witnessed the sole survivor of Flat E car-
rying a cigarette lighter and attempting to burn a piece of paper
shortly after evacuation. This man became the primary suspect.
Peter explained:

> We discovered the cigarette lighter on the footpath and that was the
> one believed to have been used to light the fire. With the aid of the
> staff we identified the likely person that lit the fire. So we identified
> him, we located him, we then put him in the care of one of the
> staff and he was seated in another building in an office, just for his
> wellbeing and so we knew where he was. I suppose he was in custody
> in a sense.[14]

Further investigations by the Victoria Police and MFB confirmed
that the most probable cause of the fire was bedding having been
set alight with a cigarette lighter. Although a resident was identified
as the perpetrator, his intellectual disability precluded any criminal
charges being laid as there was no apparent criminal intent.
Subsequently, the focus of public attention shifted towards the State
and its role in contributing to the deaths of nine men in its care.

The response to the fire from people in Australia and overseas was at times overwhelming. Letters of condolence were sent from afar and memorial services were held throughout the country. On 19 April 1996, a group of Queenslanders held a silent vigil in King George Square Brisbane. The attendees collated a signed petition that was sent to Victorian premier, Jeff Kennett, in support of existing demands for an independent Royal Commission to investigate the fire and deaths of the nine men.[15] John Kelleher, a forensic officer from the Fire and Explosion Unit of the Victoria Police, believed that the passionate community response was due to the Cottages being an iconic, State facility:

> Kew Cottages was well-known. There wouldn't be too many public facilities that are as well-known. As it was managed by the State Government, which is meant to represent *the community*, I think that many people perceived it as a community responsibility. So when the fire happened the whole community was concerned about how something like this could happen; what have *we* done wrong or what could *we* have done better?[16]

The general public were demanding answers. As a Royal Commission was never instigated, information about the fire was reliant upon investigations conducted by the Victoria Police, MFB and the Coroner's Inquest.

John Kelleher led the fire investigation on behalf of the Victoria Police. He was in attendance on the night of the blaze. By the following afternoon forensic officers had finished examining the unit. Evidence was recorded, logged and secured for future use. According to John, in many ways the fire was not complex; the cause and sequence of events appeared to be clearly evident. However, similar fires in other congregate care facilities and community demands for answers contributed to the formation of a joint fire investigation team between the Police and MFB:

> There were so many people that died that we had to try to determine whether it did actually happen the way that we suspected. It's all very well to say: 'We agree with the Fire Service, or the Fire Service agrees with us, we all agree with each other about how it started.'

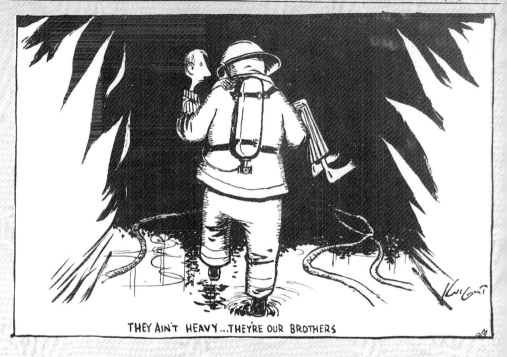

THEY AIN'T HEAVY...THEY'RE OUR BROTHERS

Popular reaction to the Kew fire. (Mark
Knight, 'They ain't heavy … they're
our brothers'. Courtesy of *Herald and
Weekly Times* Photographic Collection)

But then again we could both have been wrong! This was really
important to the community, so it was something that we wanted
to get right. There were issues too, like did the smoke detectors
work properly, do they provide adequate warning, and how long
exactly does a smoke detector take to go off, given these particular
circumstances? So there were a few questions to be answered.[17]

The joint investigation team was headed by John and Inspector Garry
Martin from the Brigade's Fire Investigation and Analysis Unit. They
conducted a series of fire tests between May and July 1996, including
a re-enactment that was staged with the full support of the Coroner.
The re-enactment was attended by members of the inquest, Victoria
Police, MFB and other interested parties. Fire personnel were onsite
in case the fire got out of control. The re-enactment was recorded for
research and as possible evidence. John recalled that this large-scale
test confirmed the speed and ferocity of the blaze:

There were around 40 to 50 people in a viewing area. Again there had to be Fire Service people in there to supervise them as it was possible that an evacuation may have been required. We're always safety-conscious but something like that could have had a lot of potential for accidents. It was a huge fire, the re-enactment … Once the fire started, I was right back in the viewing area … It was a frightening experience really, seeing how quickly it all developed. The flames were 10 or 12 metres high coming out of the building, it was really remarkable … It brought home the reality of it. You often think: 'How could you be overcome' and at Kew 'How could so many people be caught unawares?' When you realise how quickly it happens and what a violent event it is, it makes people realise how these things could have happened. It's not something that took three quarters of an hour or an hour, where people would have had plenty of warning, it was all over in a few minutes.[18]

Many people believed that the physical layout of Unit 30/31 contributed to the deaths of the nine men. In various reports and interviews, people often spoke of the men being lost inside their unit, unable to find a way out. As part of its renovation process, the unit had been partitioned into small maze-like living spaces in an attempt to provide more privacy and personalised conditions. In February 2006, fellow research team member, Chris Dew, and I inspected an identical building, Unit 28/29, which was no longer inhabited. There was a sense of eeriness as we entered the building, Chris had been here before, but this was my first time. As we started our journey into the unit, stories of the fire sprang to mind. I was trying to envisage what it must have been like for people who had been trapped inside Unit 30/31. Walking around the first section the layout seemed straightforward; we just followed the passageways. However, before long we became disoriented. The unit was divided into five flats with some interconnecting rooms and shared facilities. As we stood in a corridor wondering which way we had come from and where we needed to go next I spotted a map secured to the wall. We took this map and used it to navigate around the rest of the building. Apparently, easy navigation was not a major concern in the redevelopment of these old dormitories. Even some staff found the design challenging. Jan Sharp recalled that when, 'they put partitions up, they became like rabbit warrens; we used to go in and get lost'.[19]

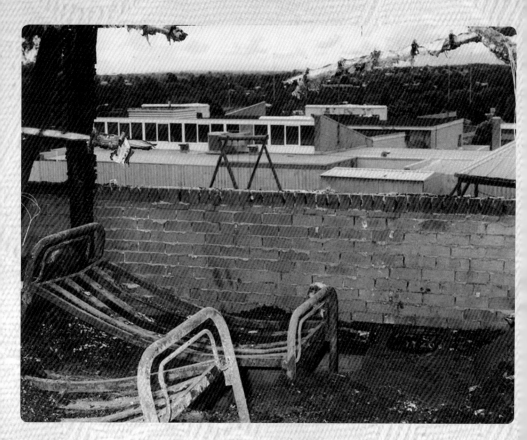

Burnt-out bedroom, Unit 31.
(Courtesy of the Victoria Police)

As part of the inquest, the Coroner and associated parties inspected the charred remains of the Unit. Ian Freckelton, counsel representing the Office of the Public Advocate at the Coroner's Inquest, was struck by the 'labyrinthine construction'.[20] The Coroner found that the building was a complex structure that created difficulties in supervision and evacuation. He also criticised building practices and materials.[21] For outsiders the physical design of Unit 30/31 appeared highly problematic, but for those living within the facility it was a familiar place many called 'home'. The discovery of Thomas, Shayne and Ronald near doorways would appear to support the fact that they knew where exits were located. Sadly, the intensity of the fire stopped them from reaching safety.

The results of the joint investigation provided critical evidence in the Coroner's Inquest and contributed to improved safety measures being implemented in State facilities across Victoria. John Kelleher also recognised that the collaborative nature of the investigation furthered positive relationships between the Victoria Police and MFB, 'as joint exercises go it was absolutely huge, we had a marvellous relationship with the Fire Service. It was a terrible thing to happen, but some good came out of it in terms of the relationship between the Police and the Fire Service, and the development of cooperative procedures.'[22] The loss of nine residents was not in vain. Although offering little comfort to those who grieved for their relatives, friends and charges, undoubtedly the lives of others in State care were better protected through improved fire safety measures which were introduced as a result of the Kew fire investigations.

The dedication of some Kew staff in caring for residents was highlighted by their efforts to save the men accommodated in Unit 30/31. When the fire alarm was raised staff in surrounding units were telephoned and, after ensuring the security of their residents, literally ran to the scene of the fire. Police witness statements revealed the determination and courage of a handful of staff who assisted in the evacuation, risking their lives by repeatedly going into the burning unit in search of residents. In particular, the Coroner commended the two night staff who were on duty, Chea Earpeng (Peng) and Bartful Frlan. Nurse, Julie Carpenter, spoke candidly about the devastating impact of the fire on Peng, 'One of the staff on duty that night, I don't think he'll ever work again in his life. He was a Cambodian refugee, he'd been through so much in his life before he came and worked at Kew. He was the loveliest person. He was so fond of the residents and he kept running back into that building trying to get them out. He had a total breakdown.'[23] Fellow staff member, Muharem Sen, who was one of the first people to help with evacuations, carried Peng out of the burning building after he collapsed from smoke inhalation. Peng was later hospitalised and treated but was permanently scarred by his experience.[24]

On 8 March 2006, unit manager, Helen Wilson, and I were seated at the kitchen table in Unit 25, recording her stories about working at Kew Cottages over the previous 33 years. We had been speaking for nearly two hours when I asked her about the 1996 fire. Immediately Helen's face turned pale; she lowered her eyes and carefully gathered her thoughts. As she started to recall her experience of the tragic event, Helen became tearful. Even 10 years after the fire, her voice quavered as she declared, 'I'm going to get upset talking about this now.'[25] Helen's response to my question was typical of most of interviewees who were questioned about this issue. Even professionals, such as police and fire officers who attended and investigated the fire, spoke about its enduring emotional impact.

Helen's anguish was evident as she recalled the scene at the Cottages on the morning after the fire:

> nothing really prepared me for what I met at the front gate … I've never experienced anything like it. There were fire trucks everywhere, there were ambulances everywhere, there were police cars everywhere. There were people stopping you from driving in. We were told not to approach that area. It was the worst thing that you can possibly imagine. Then when you're driving through it you just couldn't take your eyes off the building. I had to sort of drive around to get to the unit that I was working at then, and then to go in and all the staff, everybody was just like walking ghosts that day, honestly, yes it was just awful.[26]

Helen also took note of the residents' response:

> Some of them really understood what had actually happened, that the building had burnt down and that the people had died, that they'd been burnt and were dead. Others were sort of questioning why, what's happened there? You could just see that it had an effect on everybody, whether they understood what had happened or not, they could actually see the building and see that it was burnt. There was this real hollow feeling over Kew for weeks and weeks and weeks after that.[27]

This description of Kew immediately after the fire was echoed by many interviewees. Julie Carpenter worked in the Hospital Unit close to 30/31, but was in New Zealand when she heard about the fire. She remembered that on her return the staff were traumatised, '*everybody* was *so* affected, even people that had a really hard exterior, could not help but be affected by it'.[28] Staff and residents shared in their grief at funeral and memorial services to honour the victims of the fire. Ralph Dawson expressed sadness at the loss of his fellow residents, 'there was a fireball, I watched it on TV … One client has a cigarette lighter on his bed … but the whole unit went up, it went whoof! Like a fireball … I went to the funeral … There was one of these fire clients in the coffin … I knew I was going to cry, I had tears in my eyes. I saw the coffin going down there, I burst in tears, I couldn't *help* it.'[29]

Unlike the public who relied upon soundbites and brief descriptions published about the victims, many residents and staff had known the men, some for decades. Julie laughed as she recalled the antics of some of the deceased:

> I knew every one of those men because at some stage they'd been in the Hospital Unit, even if it was only to have their dental treatment done under anaesthetic. Because the building was so close to us we used to see them. They were always in the yard outside. Sometimes they used to throw things on our roof. One of them used to climb up on our roof … He'd run along the roof, and we'd say: 'Ronny's up on the roof again … Come on Ronny, get down off the roof.' He'd run about three more times and then he'd get down and he'd go back home.[30]

Regrettably for Ronald, 'home' was Unit 30/31.

Kew management organised for counselling to be available for staff and residents. However, most staff relied on support from one another. Some others sought alternate forms of counselling such as pastoral care from James Scannell, a Catholic priest who worked at Kew for many years. Grief and discontent felt by many staff was exacerbated by inaccurate media reportage. The media relied upon hastily gathered information and supposition to compile initial reports that were published and broadcast the morning after the fire. At first, some Kew employees openly spoke to the media in an effort to provide a more accurate account of the men's lives at Kew Cottages. Before long, staff were ordered by management not to engage in discussions with the media, but instead to direct them to the government department responsible for Kew. Many staff were upset by this order because of the misinformation being published and wanted to publicly set the record straight. Michael Glenister was one of those frustrated at false media reports. He wanted 'to come out and say the truth'.[31] Anger was directed towards the management of Kew and the department for the imposed gag.

In many ways, the Kew Cottages Parents' Association took on this advocacy role in place of staff. From the outset the Association was actively involved in gathering information, disseminating viewpoints and providing support for those affected by the fire. This support extended beyond the parents that were members of the Association to non-members, their families and staff, particularly those involved in direct care roles. For many parents, Geoffrey Welchman, the president of the Parents' Association, was a key contact after the fire. An anxious parent, Hilda Logan, was one of the first to call Geoff:

> I was in bed, and my elder sister rang me and she had just heard on the news that there was a fire at Kew Cottages. So I rang Geoff and he said he'd already had a call. I said: 'Well where is it?' He said: 'I don't know.' … I decided that I would ring our unit on the direct line and I got onto Gus Banko … Gus answered the phone and I said: 'I believe that there's a fire Gus, where is it?' He said: '30/31 and it's awful.' So I rang Geoff back and told him where it was.[32]

Shortly after Hilda's phone call, Geoff and his wife Elsie, headed for Kew to become fully apprised of the situation. A leading member of the Association, Rosalie Trower, recalled that as Geoff and Elsie drove to the Cottages they heard a radio broadcast that reported the loss of 13 lives. She stated, 'Poor old Geoff Welchman, he went straight out there with Elsie, and they said by the time he got there the tears were coming down his face, the number had jumped to 13 dead, well, it so happened it wasn't, thank God.'[33] Two years earlier,

Geoff and Elsie's son had lived in Unit 31. Undoubtedly they were shocked and contemplating what might have been. Geoff and Elsie were not alone in journeying to Kew that night. Other members of the Association arrived onsite, opening up the kiosk to provide tea and support for those in need.

The following day the Parents' Association was bombarded by requests from the media for information about the Cottages and the fire. A small group of members, Geoff Welchman, Des Lowther, Hilda Logan and Rosalie Trower, a journalist by trade, took on the responsibility of public relations. On the first morning Rosalie believed that she would be able to handle the workload, but by that evening she sought assistance:

> My sister rang me up and said: 'Would you like me to come up?' ... I said: 'No, I'll be right, don't worry.' I rang her that night and I said: 'Please come, I need somebody to make me a cup of tea.' So she came hurtling up here ... I remember one time I went out [for] ... a short time, I had 13 messages on my machine and all [from] the papers.[34]

Over the coming weeks and months the Association was pivotal in feeding information to the media. This public relations strategy kept Kew Cottages in the headlines by highlighting years of government neglect and public apathy.

For several years the Parents' Association had publicly and continually criticised the Victorian Government for budget cuts at the Cottages and for failing to meet its duty of care. Geoff Welchman spearheaded public and political campaigns to rectify the substandard conditions present at Kew, 'we were suing the government in the Supreme Court ... they weren't doing what they were bound to do under the *[Disability] Act*. We challenged them in the Supreme Court that they *must* do it.'[35] The Association was in the process of suing the Government when the fire occurred. Members believed that the 1996 fire epitomised State neglect. The media appeared to support this viewpoint and published articles about Kew with headlines such as 'Claims Quality of Life Worse than Jail'.[36] Scathing media reports often contained information and quotes provided by Association representatives.

Comments and Recommendations
into Fire and Nine Deaths at Kew Residential
Services on 8 April 1996:

1. The State of Victoria owed a duty of care to the staff and the nine intellectually disabled residents at Kew Residential Services.

2. For ten years (since 1986), the State of Victoria had been given warning after warning by consultants, experts, personnel and different government instrumentalities as to the inadequacy of the fire safety system at Kew Residential Services.

3. These warnings had been given to the State of Victoria over the period of several governments and departmental agencies having responsibilities for fire safety at Kew Residential Services.

4. The present government and the Department of Human Services had made substantial efforts to upgrade significantly the fire safety systems at Kew Residential Services.

5. However, the fact remains that ten years is far too long for the State of Victoria to have got its house in order, particularly when considering the life and safety of the persons to which it owed a duty of care.

6. The State of Victoria has contributed to the fire and deaths of the nine residents because, despite all warnings it had received over the decade from 1986, no proper fire safety system was in place at the time of the fire.

7. This is not the only way in which the State of Victoria has contributed to the deaths. These other ways are detailed in the findings.

8. The role of various consultants and contractors was comprehensively investigated during the inquest, and a number of shortcomings, areas of criticism and scope for improvement have been identified; however, on the recognised legal standard, those parties have not contributed to the deaths.

9. Nonetheless, it is encouraging that the State of Victoria was undertaking substantial efforts towards a proper fire safety upgrade at the time of the fire. In addition, during the currency of the inquest, the State has made several positive moves towards improving fire safety. The commitment of $75.5 million to 'continue the program of fire safety audits and works' in Department of Human Services facilities is a particularly positive step. The extent of the positive work towards improving fire safety along with the implementation of the many recommendations will, no doubt, significantly reduce the chance of such an event recurring.

10. Throughout the inquest, the importance of learning from the fire so that the same errors will not occur again has been stressed. The positive lessons learnt from the investigation of the fire will have consequences for other governmental and private institutions that look after intellectually or otherwise disabled persons.

11. The Kew Residential Services fire remains a tragedy for the State of Victoria and, in particular, for the victims and their families.

(Graeme Johnstone, *Inquest Findings, Comments and Recommendations into Fire and Nine Deaths at Kew Residential Services on 8 April 1996*, Melbourne, Victorian Coroner's Office, 1997, p 12.)

The inquest into the Kew fire was one of the longest Coronial Inquests in the State's history; sitting for 81 days. Although Jeff Kennett vehemently denied any wrongdoing on behalf of the State of Victoria, the Coronial Inquest confirmed allegations made in initial press reports that the fire was avoidable.[37] The Parents' Association sent representatives to the inquest each day, ensuring that families were not forgotten in this tragedy. In his published findings, the Coroner confirmed that evidence suggested that the fire was started by a resident. He did not find the resident to be criminally culpable because of the absence of intent due to intellectual disability. The State of Victoria was named as a major contributor to the deaths of the nine men for failing in its duty of care.[38] A class action by the Parents' Association against the Victorian Government was withdrawn in response to changes implemented after the fire.

Although anger, frustration and grief were immediate responses to the fire, by the time the Coroner's findings were handed down, on 17 October 1997, sadness, acceptance and optimism for the future care of remaining residents prevailed. The Victorian Government, probably pre-empting the Coroner's findings, allocated $75.5 million to continue audits of fire safety and works in facilities managed by the Department of Human Services.[39] At Kew, institutional safety procedures and equipment were drastically improved. The fire and inquest also revealed problems associated with large-scale congregate care. These were highlighted by a report submitted to the inquest by the Office of the Public Advocate. Plans for deinstitutionalisation of residents and the closure of Kew hastened. Within 10 years the number of residents living at the institution fell from 600 to 100. The 1996 Kew fire was a significant turning point in the history of Kew Cottages.

The deaths of Ronald, Adrian, Thomas, Bruce, Stanley, Alan, Shayne, Peter and Joseph will forever be remembered in a memorial erected within the landscape of Kew Cottages. This memorial will remain a permanent feature in the new suburb evolving on the former institution's site. In many respects, the Kew fire memorial symbolises a far greater loss of life at the Cottages than those who perished on 8 April. Many residents had died in less dramatic circumstances, some buried in paupers' graves with no one to mourn their loss. An epitaph for these residents will never be erected; they remain lost in the annals of history, perhaps to be uncovered and remembered by future generations. Like the nine men, some of these residents died because of the failure of various State Governments to adequately care for those housed in its institution. Overcrowding, understaffing and substandard housing not only made life difficult for residents, sometimes it was lethal.

The 1996 fire touched the hearts of so many people. It brought to the fore the neglected state of care for residents living in one of Australia's most significant institutions. The following poem was written by a relative of Peter Otis. It was a poignant acknowledgment of the apathy of many people in the general community towards those housed at Kew. The poem represented the turmoil and suffering of families directly affected by the tragedy and seems a fitting end to a chapter in history that most people simply call 'the Kew fire'.

Peter

It's just not fair
You had no chance
An innocent man-child
Whom we thought not much of
Until it was way too late.

We cannot even give you
A proper send off
In case the press crowd us in;
They won't let us grieve in peace.

Society didn't give a damn for you
When you were living
'Cause if they did
The fire wouldn't have taken you.

Disabled in a world of your own
You didn't understand danger
Ignorant bliss cost your life.

But what life did you have
In appalling conditions?
We give more to our prisoners
Who intentionally maim, harm and kill.

The sentence we gave you
Was far worse than any criminal
Yet you are the most innocent.

Peter, this is goodbye
My joy for you
Does not outweigh the sorrow for me
Grief is selfish

It's only for those left behind
You have no pain now.

No matter how you died
You are now a full person
Filled with love and happiness
Sharing eternity with Jesus Christ.

Hey Pete, give a kiss to mum for me
Our love for you both is endless,
Like the guilt we now carry
We have to live with that disability.[40]

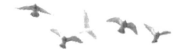

CHAPTER 11

Bye-Bye Charlie

I always believed that large style congregate care, such as Kew, wasn't the way to go. In our society, in our days it just doesn't make any sense. The community can support any of its members now, regardless of what level of need they have and you don't have to live in a big institution any more.

Charles Clark, Kew staff, 2006

Charles Clark's viewpoint reflected philosophies of deinstitutionalisation that were endorsed by many Western societies in the late 20th century. On 4 May 2001, Victorian Labor premier, Steve Bracks, announced the closure of Kew Cottages and its redevelopment into a housing estate. This decision reflected similar plans announced by Liberal premier, Jeff Kennett, in 1997. Kew's closure was a major advancement in the State's deinstitutionalisation program. At the time of Bracks' announcement, 480 residents lived onsite at Kew. Government ministers assured the public that the money raised from the sale of the Cottages was to be earmarked for the construction of community residential units for Kew residents, and remaining profits were to be diverted into disability services. Government plans stipulated that the majority of residents were to be transferred into community residential units throughout Melbourne, while 100 residents were to be allocated residences within the new housing estate.[1]

Kew's closure and redevelopment caused fierce and volatile public debate. Over several months plans were drawn and negotiated. Accusations of political money grabbing and insincerity were hurled at the Government and its supporters. In 2003, *The Age* columnist, Kenneth Davidson, referred to the plans as 'an excuse for a public land grab'.[2] This viewpoint was shared by many people in the community. In 2007, the sale of Kew Cottages was one of the key areas under investigation by the Select Committee on Public Land Development in Victoria. In dismissing Davidson's claims, the acting public advocate, Barbara Carter, argued, 'To suggest that the Kew closure is somehow different from other closures, that it is unexpected, or that it is being driven by greedy property developers, cannot be supported by any credible evidence.'[3]

Residents, staff and families were prepared for the eventual winding down of the institution. The redevelopment process suffered delays, but in 2002 the first group of residents moved away from Kew. During the next four years, 73 community residential units were built across Melbourne's suburbs and hundreds of residents were relocated. It was anticipated that by April 2008, all of the former residents would be living in their new community homes.

Some people directly associated with the Cottages responded to Government plans with trepidation, particularly families and staff members who believed that such drastic changes could have a negative impact upon residents' welfare. However, as Kew's manager, Alma Adams, recognised, continual change was a feature of life at Kew, 'One of the other things, notwithstanding that people have always lived in the one location, if you've lived at Kew what you've got used to is a lot of change. The staff change all the time, people come and go in and out of your life, clients move and clients die, they have had constant change.'[4] Many staff were also worried about the security of their employment and possible redundancies.

Other people celebrated Kew's closure as the demise of an anachronistic institution. Victoria's Minister for Community Services, from 2002–06, Sherryl Garbutt stated, 'Kew Cottages belongs to a bygone era where people with an intellectual disability were hidden from the community like a shameful secret. That is why we are closing them.'[5] The testimony of most interviewees revealed that deinstitutionalisation offered far more benefits than disadvantages.

Alma Adams was charged with the responsibility of overseeing the closure and redevelopment of Kew as she had previous experience in closing institutions such as Caloola, Janefield and Kingsbury. While intense debate raged, the residents were informed about the decision and its implications for their future. When appropriate, residents, families, guardians and/or advocates were consulted about transition plans and processes. The Office of the Public Advocate received financial support from the Department of Human Services to provide individual representation for residents who did not have a third party to advocate on their behalf. By 2003, 124 residents required such assistance.[6] The Office also served as an independent body that monitored the redevelopment process to ensure that peoples' rights were protected.

In planning for residents' relocation, some families requested that their relatives remain onsite. In 2005, Mary Scully was determined that her brother Michael be housed in a community residential unit as part of the new estate:

> I have always stated that I want Michael to stay onsite, at Kew, my parents asked for that … 'Fight for him to stay on the site for life' and that's what I'm doing. I think Michael has a right to stay onsite, he's done a lot for Kew, in his way, by the Tipping Appeal. It has been his home for 50 years, why can't it be his home for the rest of his life?[7]

It was Michael's story of being tied to a stake in his backyard that triggered the 1953 Tipping Appeal which raised significant funds to improve the living conditions at the Cottages (see Chapter 8). Mary was unsuccessful in her bid. Rosalie Trower, in contrast, was victorious in her fight for her son, Stephen, to be allocated a house at Kew:

> I went into this room, where there were a lot of bureaucrats sitting
> around, clever people, and of course they said … 'Where would you
> like Steve to live, Rosalie?' I said: 'Kew Cottages site.' 'No he can't *do*
> that' [they said]. I said: 'It may not be *your* option, but it is *my* option
> for *my* son.' Well then the arguments started, and this went on for
> months. 'Look we've got lovely land at Glen Waverley, Steve would
> be *closer* to you, and it'll be easier for you to get to him.' I said: 'Hold
> it there, this is not what's best for me, it's what I consider is best for
> my son and I would suggest I know him better than you people do.'
> In the end they gave up.[8]

When plans were being drawn up for residents' relocation, the Kew
Cottages Parents' Association proposed onsite cluster housing. In
1991–92, the Association had lobbied the Victorian Government
to sell off a portion of Kew's land and build a cluster-style housing
estate for residents. This idea was rejected. When the 2001 closure
was announced, the proposal re-emerged. However, the Government
and many other people in the community were concerned that such
a development would perpetuate the segregation of Kew residents
from mainstream society. Rosalie Trower was critical of this
viewpoint. She believed that a 'community' existed at Kew which
was worth preserving, 'there's a great deal of talk around these days
… about developing communities, *this was our community*, and
it's all taken away from us now and it's very sad'.[9] In her response
to Kenneth Davidson's assertion that parents inherently spoke
in the best interests of their children and that they wanted cluster
housing, Barbara Carter wrote 'Leaving aside the issue of whether
the preferences of family can be seen as synonymous with the wishes
of the people actually living there, a "choice" for institutional/village
type housing in these circumstances results in a lack of choice in
the everyday matters that the rest of us take for granted – meals,
outings, friends and other pleasures of life.'[10] Cluster housing was
again rejected by the Government.

One of the extraordinary stories that emerged from Kew's
redevelopment was the proactive efforts of one group of parents,
spearheaded by Hilda Logan, to ensure the best possible rehousing outcome for their children. Hilda was a leading member of the

Parents' Association and endorsed the cluster housing concept. When it failed, she was anxious to secure her son's future:

> Once we lost the fight I couldn't see the sense in beating my breast ... My son went to live at Narre Warren. Funnily enough I copped quite a lot of flack from some of the parents. I don't know why, I think some of them saw me as having given up the fight for my son to remain at Kew, but I'd never ever said that I was particularly enamoured for him to remain at Kew once things were moving on.[11]

Hilda located a plot of land that she considered to be perfect for a community residential unit. She approached long time friends, including Association members Geoffrey and Elsie Welchman, as to whether they would join her in lobbying the Government to appropriate the land and build a residential unit for their sons. In the end, Hilda generated support from four other Kew families.

United, they approached the Victorian Government. Geoff stated 'Hilda Logan found the spot there and we fought with the Department to bid for it ... [we] got very close to losing it altogether, but with Hilda as the secretary of the Parents' Association and your's truly as the president, we managed to influence them ... Then they built the house, it's a luxurious place, much better than he ever had at Kew, that's for sure.'[12] Hilda explained that the major reason she sourced land in Narre Warren was for her son to be cared for in the community by a trusted member of the Kew staff, 'I'll tell you the real reason why I was after that land. My son has had one of the best carers in the Cottages looking after him for years, his name is Alf Barta, and some of the cheeky staff at Kew referred to him as "my other son" and guess where Alf Barta lives? ... Narre Warren ... and Alf works in the house.'[13] Even though there were no guarantees that Alf was going to be assigned to work in that particular community house, Hilda was willing to take the chance.

In 2005, the Narre Warren house was officially opened. This group of parents were overjoyed with their success. Hilda stated, 'I think that life is better for them in a house ... I think that they like where they live and the house is lovely, it's a happy house.'[14] Elsie Welchman was content with her son David's reaction to community living, 'he expresses himself a lot more since he went into the house than he ever did'.[15] Hilda was surprised that more families were not proactive. However, the thought of engaging in the relocation process in this manner probably never crossed the minds of most people. In addition, several families who had relatives at Kew were elderly and/or lived in remote areas which made this task virtually impossible.

While the majority of residents appear to have benefited from deinstitutionalisation, a very small number have struggled to successfully make the transition. In 2006, Alma Adams noted:

> We've had one client who has some very significant transitional issues, he also had times here when he had very real difficulties as well, so maybe it was coincidental, maybe not, but he certainly had very difficult transition issues. There are another couple of people who also found it a bit difficult moving, but we've now got well over 365 people who haven't.[16]

One reason for the difficulties may have been due to the fact that most residents had not spent substantial periods of time away from the institution.

Before the redevelopment, residents' contact with the community mostly involved brief encounters with the outside world. A minority of Kew residents, such as Ted Rowe, Patrick Reed and Lois Philmore, had been actively supported to move away from the institution. Former chief executive officer, Max Jackson also noted:

> even before the notion of deinstitutionalisation was coined, we were moving people out, not in huge numbers, but through our Social Work Department where opportunities were available either to move older people into nursing homes or to relocate some clients back with their families or semi-independent living.[17]

Gradually, through the provision of freedom of movement, day programs, excursions and holidays, residents increasingly experienced life beyond the institution. Raymond Bouker looked forward to going to the football to see his team, Richmond, play 'I go to the football with my brother ... Paul, and Paul's wife as well.'[18] Hundreds of residents also stayed at a holiday home purchased by the Parents'

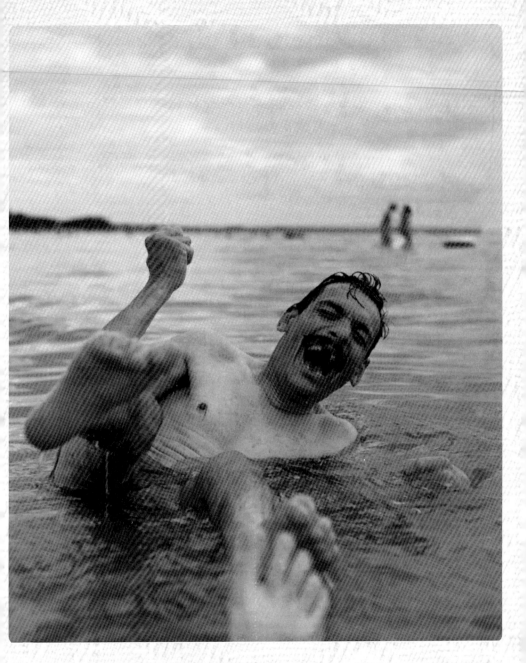

A resident enjoying a day at the
beach, circa 1990s. (Courtesy of Kew
Residential Services, Department of
Human Services, Victoria)

Association in 1983 at Tootgarook. Resident, Wendy Pennycuick, enjoyed her holidays at the beach with best friend Robyn:

CORINNE   Have you ever been to Tootgarook?

WENDY   Yes we have, take in turns … every year.

CORINNE   Who would you go down with?

WENDY   The staff, and … Robyn goes … We sleep in and go on outings.[19]

These experiences gave residents a taste of life outside of the Cottages. However, they were distinct, short events which did not replicate long term community living.

The rehousing scheme devised for Kew's closure recognised this problem and programs were introduced to ensure that residents were an active part of the transition process. Some attended meetings, proposed potential housemates, visited the site where their houses were to be built and chose décor for their bedrooms. Donald Starick was pleased to select furniture for his bedroom, 'New bed … Brown colour.'[20]

Moving away from Kew resulted in sacrifices being made by some residents. For a select group of residents, who were ambulant and mobile, one of the major losses was their freedom to socialise and move around independently. Patty Rodgers noted that in the community she was unable to walk around her neighbourhood without being accompanied by staff.[21] David Honner longed for his friends who had been relocated, 'I miss them a lot.'[22] In community residential units, most residents are reliant upon staff to ensure that friendship networks are maintained. The ability of staff to fulfil this function heavily relies upon their knowledge of residents' relationships and their willingness to offer active support.

The story of Barry Evans highlights the negative experiences of community living encountered by a few residents. Barry was assigned a place in a community residential unit that housed a group of people who exhibited challenging behaviours. His first experience of deinstitutionalisation was somewhat distressing:

BARRY I didn't like it ... It was just too rough, I reckoned it was too rough ... Liam Ford, he was too rough for me ... Oh he was nasty.

CORINNE Did he hurt you?

BARRY Yes.

CORINNE What did he do?

BARRY Gave me two black eyes.[23]

Unhappy living in the community, Barry moved back to Kew. Despite his previous difficulties, Barry has accepted that he will have to adjust to life in a community residential unit. Staff are aware of his history and offer him guidance and assistance when necessary.

Many residents were relieved and excited about the move from Kew. This was poignantly highlighted in recollections about the reactions of former residents upon hearing the word 'Kew' or returning to the institution. One community visitor claimed that mentioning 'Kew' to some former residents was akin to discussing 'the war' with traumatised veterans. She recalled that on a visit to a community residential unit:

> I mentioned 'the war' ... I mentioned 'Kew' and the man went to his room, he was so distressed ... when I went to his room to check on him, he was hitting the bed head saying to me, 'Not Kew, not Kew, not Kew, not Kew.'[24]

Michael Glenister also witnessed this type of response among residents in his community house. Michael recalled that a few weeks after moving from Kew the residents returned to the Cottages to collect an item from one of the units. He was surprised by the fervent reaction of residents:

> the staff took the guys off in the bus and they came back and they started saying to me: 'Oh, gee, you should have heard it, going round the roundabout at Kew, there was all this commotion from the back and all these cries of: "I don't want to be here", [or that] sort of thing.' And I thought: 'Oh, that's interesting, but I'll take that with a

grain of salt, I didn't see it myself'... So I set the residents up. I went out and started to speak to them and I said: 'Oh well, I hear you guys really liked Kew today so we'll move back there.' And one of the residents goes: 'No, no, no! ... We're not going back to Kew, we live in a house now!' And it blew me away.[25]

Michael noted that he was taken aback because when the protesting resident lived at Kew she was, 'the smartest one in their unit, had the freedom to roam wherever they wanted and do what they wanted'.[26]

The reaction of many residents to the closure of Kew and their subsequent rehousing was extremely optimistic. In 1999, Patty Rodgers was relocated into a community residential unit. When I asked her what she thought about Kew Cottages and leaving she replied, 'I don't like it ... I just I hate it ... I'm happy to get out of Kew.'[27] Raymond Bouker reported that when the last group of residents left the Cottages to be rehoused in offsite community residential units they waved and shouted 'Bye-Bye Charlie!'[28] These sentiments were echoed by many Kew residents. One exception was David Honner, who stated that he was saddened by Kew's demise, 'I'm not happy about it closing ... Oh well, what can you do? They're closing, and what can you do?'[29] However, he did say that he was looking forward to moving into an onsite community residential unit, 'I'm a little bit happy about it.'[30] When I asked residents about leaving the Cottages the word they used frequently to describe the transition was 'happy'. Ralph Dawson's comments about community living reflected the attitude of most resident interviewees, 'I'm very happy here ... I've got my keys and my own bedroom ... No more sharing.'[31] Although community residential units have a specific set of care issues, such as the potential for them to become 'mini-institutions', many of Kew's former residents prefer the personalised care and philosophy of active support in the houses. Raymond Bouker remarked, 'I like it better here.'[32]

At Kew, the ability of many residents to live an enjoyable life had been stifled by the oppressive nature of large-scale institutional care. As Kew Cottages is progressively dismantled and new houses emerge from the rubble, one can only hope that the deprivations that many residents suffered at the Cottages are counterbalanced by high quality levels of community care which has been promised by the Victorian Government. For as academic David Hopkins has noted, 'Given the right conditions people with significant disabilities can achieve outstanding outcomes.'[33]

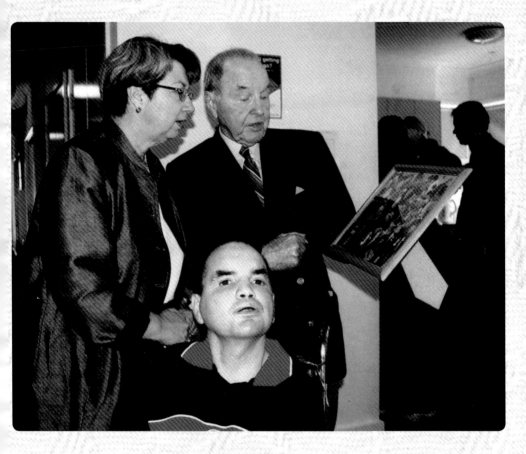

Front: Paul Westgarth.
Back: Minister for Community Services,
Sherryl Garbutt and Bill Westgarth (Paul's
father), at the official opening of Paul's
community residential unit, 2003.
(Courtesy of Kew Residential Services,
Department of Human Services, Victoria)

Notes

Introduction

1 Colin Barnes and Geoff Mercer, *Disability*, Cambridge, UK, Polity Press, 2003, pp 27–28.

2 'Report of the Inspector of Asylums on the Hospitals for the Insane for the Year 1887', *Victorian Parliamentary Papers*, Session 1888, vol 3, Appendix C, p 44.

3 Wilfrid Brady, 'The *Mental Health Act* (Victoria) 1962, *Australian Children Limited*', vol 1, no 7 (October 1963), p 345.

4 Kelley Johnson and Rannveig Traustadóttir (eds), *Deinstitutionalization and People with Intellectual Disabilities: In and Out of Institutions*, London, Jessica Kingsley Publishers, 2005, p 19.

5 Interview with Ralph Dawson, 3 August 2006.

Part I: The Journey to Kew

1 Interview with Patrick Reed, 21 March 2006; interview with Barry Evans, 26 July 2006.

2 Interview with James Barry Woods, 8 September 2006.

3 Interview with Andrew Ledwidge, 31 August 2006.

Chapter 1: A River of Tears

1 'A Country Mother', Letter to the Editor, *Herald*, 5 October 1948, p 4.

2 Ibid.

3 Ibid. The term 'Mongol' was often used to refer to a child with Down Syndrome. This was based on the belief that the children looked like people from Mongolia (who were mistakenly assumed to have had arrested development). The term was discredited in the 1960s.

4 A history of ultrasound, amniocentesis and chorionic villus sampling can be found at the following webpages: <http://www.ob-ultrasound.net/amniocentesis.html> and <http://www.ob-ultrasound.net/history1.html> (last accessed 10 January 2008).

5 Interview with George and Olive Earl, 5 June 2006; interview with James and Anna Davison, 15 March 2006.

6 Interview with Rose Miller, 7 March 2006.

7 Interview with James and Anna Davison.

8 Interview with Fran van Brummelen, 30 August 2005.

9 Arthur Lloyd, *Payment By Results: Kew Cottages First 100 Years 1887–1987*, Melbourne, Kew Cottages and

St Nicholas Parents' Association Inc, 1987, pp 105–11.

10 Interview with Rose Miller.

11 Interview with William (Bill) Westgarth, 19 January 2006.

12 Joan Jones, 'Paper Presented at the Third Annual General Meeting of the Kew Cottages Historical Society', Melbourne, unpublished manuscript, Kew Cottages Historical Society, 23 May 1990.

13 Ibid.

14 Ibid.

15 Ibid.

16 Interview with James and Anna Davison.

17 Ibid.

18 Ibid.

19 Ibid.

20 Ibid.

21 Interview with George and Olive Earl.

22 Ibid.

23 Ibid.

24 Ibid.

25 Ibid.

26 Ibid.

27 Ibid.

28 Interview with Hilda Logan, 20 March 2006.

29 Ibid

30 Ibid.

31 Ibid.

32 Ibid.

33 Interview with Rosalie Trower, 21 June 2006.

34 Ibid.

35 Ibid.

36 Ibid.

37 Ibid

38 Ibid.

39 Ibid.

40 Interview with Geoffrey (Geoff) and Elsie Welchman, 11 January 2006.

41 Ibid.

42 Ibid.

43 Ibid.

44 Ibid.

45 Ibid.

46 Interview with Bill Westgarth.

47 Ibid.

48 Ibid.

49 Ibid.

50 Ibid.

51 Ibid.

52 Interview with Rose Miller.

53 Ibid.

54 Ibid.

55 Interview with Hilda Logan.

56 Interview with Rose Miller.

Chapter 2: Welcome Strangers

1 'The Village of the Damned', *The Age*, 12 April 1975.

2 Ibid.

3 *Village of the Damned*, Wolf Rilla (director) 1960.

4 Chris Paris, *Housing Australia*, Melbourne, Macmillan Education Australia Pty Ltd, 1993, p 117.

5 Sylvia Babic, 'Memoirs', unpublished manuscript, Kew Cottages Historical Society, 1988, p 5; Sylvia Babic, 'Written Submission', Kew Cottages History Project, La Trobe University, 2006, p 1.

6 Interview with Sylvia Babic, 18 January 2006.

7 Babic, 'Memoirs', p 10.

8 Interview with Kurt and Maria Kraushofer, 28 March 2006.

9 Ibid.

10 A James Hammerton and Alistair Thomson, *Ten Pound Poms: Australia's Invisible Migrants*, Manchester, Manchester University Press, 2005, pp 30–31.

11 'Report of the Director of Mental Hygiene for the Year Ended 31st December, 1948', Department of Mental Hygiene, *Victorian Parliamentary Papers*, vol 1, no 17, 1949, p 17.

12 Interview with Kurt and Maria Kraushofer.

13 Interview with Saral Nathaniel, 27 October 2005.

14 Interview with Ruth Anghie, 27 March 2006.

15 Ibid.

16 Ibid.

17 Interview with Helen Wilson, 8 March 2006.

18 Ibid.

19 Ibid.

20 Interview with David Pitt, 19 September 2005.

21 Ibid.

22 Ibid; David Buxton Pitt, *For the Love of the Children: My Life and Medical Career*, Melbourne, Pitt Publishing, 1999, p 16.

23 Interview with David Pitt.

24 Interview with Malcolm Macmillan, 9 March 2006.

25 Interview with Michael Glenister, 15 November 2005.

26 Interview with Alma Adams, 14 August 2006.

27 See Victorian Government Department of Human Services <http://www.dhs.vic.gov.au/ kewredevelopment>. See also Kew Cottages Coalition <http://www. kew.org.au> for an alternative point of view. Websites were last accessed on 10 January 2008.

28 Interview with Val Smorgon, 23 April 2006.

29 Ibid.

Chapter 3: Beyond 'Fairyland'

1 Jeannette Hodgkinson (née Brady), 'A Few Memories of the Children's Cottages', Kew Cottages History Project, La Trobe University, 24 January 2007.

2 Interview with Philip Brady, 9 November 2006.

3 Hodgkinson.

4 Interview with Bill Westgarth, 19 January 2006.

5 Interview with Lois Philmore, 25 January 2007.

6 Astrid Judge, 'Reflections, Memories and Sources: Growing Up at Kew Cottages', Health and History, vol 9, issue 1 (2007), par 23, <http://www. historycooperative.org/journals/ hah/9.1/judge.html> (last accessed 10 January 2008).

7 Interview between Cliff Judge and Ted Wilson, circa 1987, Kew Cottages Historical Society.

8 Austra Kurzeme, 'Written Recollection of Kew Cottages by Sister Kurzeme', unpublished manuscript, Kew Cottages Historical Society, circa 1987, p 2.

9 Interview between Fran van Brummelen and Austra Kurzeme, 3 September 1987, Kew Cottages Historical Society.

10 Interview with Patrick Reed, 3 August 2007.

11 Interview with Edward (Ted) Rowe, 20 April 2006.

12 Sylvia Babic, 'Written Submission', Kew Cottages History Project, La Trobe University, 2006, pp 11–12.

13 Interview between Fran van Brummelen and Austra Kurzeme, 10 September 1987, Kew Cottages Historical Society.

14 Interview with Ralph Dawson, 3 August 2006.

15 Dianne Pymble, 'Written Recollections', Kew Cottages History Project, La Trobe University, 22 September 2006.

16 Kurzeme, 'Written Recollection', p 8.

17 Interview with Ted Rowe.

18 Interview with Patrick Reed.

19 Interview with Philip Brady.

20 Interview with Ralph Dawson.

21 Interview with David Honner, 12 April 2007.

22 Interview with David Sykes, 16 October 2006.

23 'Lone Junior Nurse's 44 Asylum "Children"', Truth, 17 April 1937, p 11.

24 'Report of the Mental Hygiene Authority for the Year Ended 31 December, 1960', Victorian Parliamentary Papers, vol 2, p 80.

25 Interview with John (Jack) and Margaret Cotter, 6 March 2006.

26 Ibid.

27 'Probe into Crowding at Kew Cottages', Progress Press, 1 November 1989.

28 Interview between Cliff Judge and Ted Wilson.

29 Interview with Ted Rowe.

30 Mark Rapley, The Social Construction of Intellectual Disability, Cambridge, UK, Cambridge University Press, 2004, pp 46–47; Cliff Judge and Fran van Brummelen, Kew Cottages: The World of Dolly Stainer, Melbourne, Spectrum Publications, 2002, pp 41–49.

31 Interview between Cliff Judge and Ted Wilson.

32 Interview with Jack and Margaret Cotter.

33 Interview with Ruth Anghie, 27 March 2006.

34 Interview with Ted Rowe.

35 Interview with Jack and Margaret Cotter.

36 Interview with Kurt and Maria Kraushofer, 28 March 2006.

37 Interview between Julie McInnes and Evelyn Richards, September 1987, Kew Cottages Historical

Society.
38 Interview with Lois Philmore.
39 Interview with Kurt and Maria Kraushofer.
40 Ibid.
41 Interview with Nick Konstantaras, 15 June 2006.
42 Bengt Nirje, 'The Normalization Principle and its Human Management Implications', in Robert Kugel and Wolf Wolfensberger (eds), *Changing Patterns in Residential Services for the Mentally Retarded*, Washington, President's Committee on Mental Retardation, 1969, p 181; Wolf Wolfensberger, *Normalization: The Principle of Normalization in Human Services*, Toronto, National Institute on Mental Retardation, 1972.
43 Interview with Alma Adams, 14 August 2006.
44 Interview with John Wakefield, 15 March 2006.
45 Interview with Christine Walton, 27 February 2006.

Chapter 4: 'No Buttons, No Braces and No Laces!'

1 Interview with Ralph Dawson, 6 August 2007.
2 Interview with Raymond Bouker, 6 September 2006.
3 Interview with Edward (Ted) Rowe, 20 April 2006.
4 Sylvia Babic, 'Memoirs', unpublished manuscript, Kew Cottages Historical Society, 1988, p 17.
5 Interview with John Wakefield, 15 March 2006.
6 Austra Kurzeme, 'Written Recollection of Kew Cottages by Sister Kurzeme', unpublished manuscript, Kew Cottages Historical Society, circa 1987, p 1.
7 Ibid., p 2.
8 Interview with Helen Wilson, 8 March 2006.
9 Interview with Eric Cunningham Dax, 9 January 2006.
10 Ibid; Eric Cunningham Dax, *Asylum to Community: The Development of the Mental Hygiene Service in Victoria, Australia*, Melbourne, FW Cheshire, 1961, p 125.
11 Interview with Kurt and Maria Kraushofer, 28 March 2006.
12 Interview with Ted Rowe.

13 Interview with Patrick Reed, 21 March 2006.
14 Interview between Fran van Brummelen and Irene Harvey, 17 August 1987, Kew Cottages Historical Society.
15 Ibid.
16 Interview between Fran van Brummelen and Austra Kurzeme, 10 September 1987, Kew Cottages Historical Society.
17 Cliff Judge and Fran van Brummelen, *Kew Cottages: The World of Dolly Stainer*, Melbourne, Spectrum Publications, 2002, p 129.
18 Interview with Kurt and Maria Kraushofer.
19 Ibid.
20 Interview with Michael Glenister, 15 November 2005.
21 Focus Group with Community Visitors, 20 June 2006.
22 Interview with Steven Wears, 7 June 2007.
23 Focus Group with Community Visitors.
24 Interview with Ralph Dawson.
25 Dax, *Asylum to Community*, pp 124–25.
26 Interview with Julie Carpenter, 24 January 2006.
27 Erving Goffman, *Asylums: Essays on the Social Situation of Mental Patients and Other Inmates*, New York, Anchor Books, 1961, pp 19–20.
28 Interview with Ted Rowe.
29 Ibid.
30 Ibid.
31 Interview between Cliff Judge and Ted Wilson, circa 1987, Kew Cottages Historical Society.
32 Ibid.
33 Focus Group with Community Visitors.
34 Interview between Cliff Judge and Margaret McDonald, circa 1987, Kew Cottages Historical Society.
35 Interview with Ruth Anghie, 27 March 2006.
36 Interview with Max Jackson, 25 January 2006.
37 Interview with Helen Wilson.
38 Interview with Patrick Reed.
39 Interview with Kurt and Maria Kraushofer.
40 Interview with Jan Sharp, 10 January 2006.

Chapter 5: Shepherd's Pie to Stir Fry

1 Interview with Edward (Ted) Rowe, 20 April 2006.
2 Reginald Ellery, *The Cow Jumped Over the Moon: Private Papers of a Psychiatrist*, Melbourne, FW Cheshire, 1956, p 139.
3 Interview with Ruth Anghie, 27 March 2006.
4 Interview with Jan Sharp, 17 January 2006.
5 Interview between Cliff Judge and Ted Wilson, circa 1987, Kew Cottages Historical Society.
6 Sylvia Babic, 'Memoirs', unpublished manuscript, Kew Cottages Historical Society, 1988, p 18.
7 Interview with Ted Rowe.
8 Interview with Eric Cunningham Dax, 9 January 2006.
9 Interview with Clare Turner, 5 August 2005.
10 Interview with Ted Rowe.
11 Ibid.
12 Ibid.
13 Interview between Fran van Brummelen and Irene Harvey, 17 August 1987, Kew Cottages Historical Society.
14 Ibid.
15 Interview with Patrick Reed, 21 March 2006.
16 Interview between Julie McInnes and Evelyn Richards, September 1987, Kew Cottages Historical Society.
17 Interview with Nick Konstantaras, 15 June 2006.
18 Interview with Wendy Pennycuick, 4 August 2007.
19 Interview with Kurt and Maria Kraushofer, 28 March 2006.
20 Interview with Andrew Ledwidge, 31 August 2006.
21 Focus Group with Community Visitors, 20 June 2006.
22 Interview with David Pitt, 19 September 2005; David Pitt, *For the Love of the Children: My Life and Medical Career*, Melbourne, Pitt Publishing, 1999, p 160.
23 Interview with David Pitt.
24 Pitt, *For the Love of the Children*, p 161.
25 Interview with Ruth Anghie.
26 Ibid.
27 Ibid.
28 Ibid.
29 Interview with Julie Carpenter, 24 January 2006.
30 Interview with Max Jackson, 25 January 2006.
31 Ibid.
32 Ibid.
33 'Pledge to Rectify Food Situation at Cottages', *Progress Press*, 27 March 1991, p 3.
34 Rosalie Trower, 'Kew Daily Food Allowance Less than for Prison', Letter to the Editor, *The Age*, 20 April 1995.
35 Interview with Michael Glenister, 13 December 2005.

Chapter 6: At the Heart of Kew's History

1 Interviews with Edward (Ted) Rowe, 20 April 2006 and 23 May 2006.
2 Interview with Lois Philmore, 25 January 2007.
3 Interviews with Patrick Reed, 21 March 2006, 5 April 2006 and 3 August 2007.
4 Interviews with David Honner, 12 April 2007 and 4 August 2007.
5 Interviews with Raymond Bouker, 14 August 2006 and 6 September 2006.
6 Interviews with Wendy Pennycuick, 19 December 2006 and 4 August 2007.
7 Interviews with Steven Wears, 24 June 2006 and 7 June 2007.
8 Interview with Patricia (Patty) Rodgers, 29 June 2006.
9 Interviews with Ralph Dawson, 3 August 2006 and 6 August 2007.
10 Interviews with John Goddard, 29 May 2006, 1 June 2006 and 8 June 2006.
11 Interviews with Andrew Ledwidge, 31 August 2006 and 26 October 2006.
12 Interviews with Donald Starick, 21 June 2006 and 6 December 2006.
13 Interview with Nick Konstantaras, 15 June 2006.
14 Interviews with James Barry Woods, 8 September 2006 and 15 September 2006; personal files held by the Victorian Department of Human Services.

Chapter 7: 'Chattel Slaves'?

1　'Caught in Kew Mincing Machine', *Truth*, 27 February 1937.

2　JP Doherty, '4431 Children's Cottages, Kew', in *Vision and Realisation: A Centenary History of State Education in Victoria*, vol 3, Education Department of Victoria, 1973, p 471.

3　Interview with Edward (Ted) Rowe, 20 April 2006.

4　Department of Mental Hygiene, 'Report of the Director of Mental Hygiene for the Year Ended 31st December 1950', *Victorian Parliamentary Papers*, vol 2, p 6.

5　Kay McCulloch, 'Kew Special School – 100 Years of Caring', *VTU Journal*, 10 December 1987, p 10.

6　Cliff Judge and Fran van Brummelen, *Kew Cottages: The World of Dolly Stainer*, Richmond, Spectrum Publications, 2002, pp 82–87.

7　Interview between Julie McInnes and Evelyn Richards, September 1987, Kew Cottages Historical Society.

8　McCulloch, p 10.

9　Interview with Andrew Ledwidge, 31 August 2006.

10　Interview with Raymond Bouker, 6 September 2006.

11　Interview with Andrew Ledwidge, 26 October 2006.

12　Interview with Raymond Bouker.

13　Maxwell Jones, *Therapeutic Community*, New York, Basic Books, 1953; Judge and van Brummelen, p 166.

14　'Report of the Mental Hygiene Authority for the Year Ended 30th June, 1955', *Victorian Parliamentary Papers*, vol 2, 1955–56.

15　'Report of the Mental Hygiene Authority for the Year Ended 31st December, 1960', *Victorian Parliamentary Papers*, vol 2, 1961–62, p 77; 'Report of the Mental Health Authority for the Period 1st January, 1964 to 31st December, 1965', *Victorian Parliamentary Papers*, vol 2, 1967, p 101; 'Report of the Mental Health Authority for the Year Ended 31st December, 1970', *Victorian Parliamentary Papers*, vol 2, 1971–72, p 81.

16　'Children's Cottages Kew: A Training Centre for the Intellectually Handicapped', brochure, np, circa 1960s.

17　'Report of the Mental Hygiene Authority for the Year Ended 30th June, 1955', *Victorian Parliamentary Papers*, vol 2, 1955–56, p 56; 'Children's Cottages Kew' brochure.

18　For information on play therapy see Virginia Axline, *Play Therapy: The Inner Dynamics of Childhood*, Cambridge, Mass, Houghton Mifflin, 1947.

19　Interviews with Andrew Ledwidge, 31 August 2006 and 26 October 2006.

20　Interview with Andrew Ledwidge, 26 October 2006.

21　Interview with John Goddard, 29 May 2006; interview with David Honner, 4 August 2007.

22　Interview with Wendy Pennycuick, 4 August 2007.

23　Interview with Clare Turner, 5 August 2005.

24　Ibid.

25　Interview with Jan Sharp, 10 January 2006.

26　Interview with Saral Nathaniel, 27 October 2005.

27　Interview with Kurt and Maria Kraushofer, 28 March 2006.

28　Interview with Max Jackson, 25 January 2006.

29　Ibid.

30　Interview with Alma Adams, 14 August 2006.

31　Ibid.

32　Interview with Ralph Dawson, 5 September 2006.

33　Interview with Hilda Logan, 20 March 2006.

34　Andrew Slevin, '"It's Times like These we Learn to Live Again"', written submission to Kew Cottages History Project, La Trobe University, 2006.

35　Ibid.

36　Interview with Ted Rowe.

37　Judge and van Brummelen, pp 139–40.

38　Quoted in 'Caught in Kew Mincing Machine', *Truth*, 27 February 1937.

39　Ibid.

40　'Report of the Mental Hygiene Authority for the Year Ended 30 June, 1953', *Victorian*

Parliamentary Papers, vol 2, p 16; 'Report of the Mental Health Authority for the Year Ended 31st December, 1968', *Victorian Parliamentary Papers*, vol 2, p 76.

41 Interview with Ted Rowe.

42 Ibid.

43 Interview with Patricia (Patty) Rodgers, 29 June 2006.

44 Interview with Wendy Pennycuick, 19 December 2006.

45 Interview with Raymond Bouker.

46 Ibid.

47 Jeannette Hodgkinson, 'A Few Memories of the Children's Cottages', written submission, Kew Cottages History Project, La Trobe University, 24 January 2007.

48 Interview with Lois Philmore, 25 January 2007.

49 Interviews with Ralph Dawson, 5 September 2006 and 6 August 2007.

50 Joan Jones, 'Paper Presented at the Third Annual General Meeting of the Kew Cottages Historical Society', Melbourne, unpublished manuscript, Kew Cottages Historical Society, 23 May 1990; Judge and van Brummelen, p 79.

51 Joan Jones.

52 Interview with Lois Philmore.

53 Interview with Nick Konstantaras, 15 June 2006.

54 Interview with Andrew Ledwidge, 26 October 2006.

55 Interview with Patrick Reed, 21 March 2006.

56 Ibid.

57 Interview with John Wakefield, 15 March 2006.

58 Transcript reading with Patrick Reed, 5 April 2006; meeting with Patrick Reed, 17 May 2007.

Chapter 8: Happy Memories?

1 Erving Goffman, *Asylums: Essays on the Social Situation of Mental Patients and Other Inmates*, New York, Anchor Books, 1961.

2 Interview with Ralph Dawson, 3 August 2006.

3 *Kew News*, April 2003, p 2.

4 Interview with Kurt and Maria Kraushofer, 28 March 2006.

5 Tom Shakespeare, Kath Gillespie-Sells and Dominic Davies, *The Sexual Politics of Disability: Untold Desires*, London, Cassell, 1996, pp 153–54.

6 Interview with Steven Wears, 7 June 2007.

7 Interview with David Honner, 4 August 2007.

8 Ibid.

9 Interview with Patty Rodgers, 29 June 2006.

10 Transcript reading with Clare Turner, 10 April 2006.

11 Interview with Fran van Brummelen, 30 August 2005.

12 Interview with John (Jack) and Margaret Cotter, 6 March 2006.

13 Ibid.

14 Interview with Fran van Brummelen.

15 Interview with Helen Wilson, 8 March 2006.

16 Interview with Hilda Logan, 20 March 2006.

17 Ibid.

18 Transcript reading with Patrick Reed, 5 April 2006.

19 Interview with Ruth Anghie, 27 March 2006.

20 Notes from a meeting with Ralph Dawson, 19 February 2007.

21 Eric Cunningham Dax, *Asylum to Community: The Development of the Mental Hygiene Service in Victoria, Australia*, Melbourne, FW Cheshire, 1961, p 89.

22 Interview with Eric Cunningham Dax, 9 January 2006.

23 Interview with Jan Sharp, 10 January 2006.

24 Interview with Steven Wears.

25 Interview with Robyn Cook, 1 March 2006.

26 Interview with Jan Sharp.

27 Arthur Lloyd, *Payment By Results: Kew Cottages First 100 Years 1887–1987*, Melbourne, Kew Cottages and St Nicholas Parents' Association Inc, 1987, p 99.

28 Interview with Jan Sharp.

29 Interview with John Goddard, 29 May 2006.

30 Interview with Robyn Cook.

31 Louise Godwin and Catherine Wade, *Kew Cottages Parents' Association: The First Fifty Years*, Melbourne, Kew Cottages Parents' Association Inc, 2007, pp 2–3.

32 Interview with Andrew Ledwidge, 31 August 2006.

33 Interview with Patty Rodgers.
34 Jeannette Hodgkinson, 'A Few Memories of the Children's Cottages', written submission, Kew Cottages History Project, La Trobe University, 24 January 2007.
35 Interview with Patrick Reed, 21 March 2006.
36 Interview with Andrew Ledwidge, 26 October 2006.
37 Interview with Patrick Reed.
38 Interview with Jack and Margaret Cotter.
39 Interview with Edward (Ted) Rowe, 20 April 2006.
40 Ibid.
41 Ibid.
42 Interview with Donald Starick, 6 December 2006.
43 Interview with John Foster, 10 October 2006.
44 Interview with Christine Walton, 27 February 2006.
45 Interview between Julie McInnes and Evelyn Richards, September 1987, Kew Cottages Historical Society.
46 Interview with Geoffrey and Elsie Welchman, 11 January 2006.
47 EW Tipping, 'The Story of 6-year-old Michael Who was Tied to a Stake', *Herald*, 6 April 1953.
48 Interview with Mary Scully, 23 August 2005.
49 EW Tipping, 'Why Michael Has Not Run Away', *Herald*, 7 April 1953.
50 EW Tipping, 'There's a Lot to be Done Yet at Kew', *Herald*, 2 October 1954.
51 EW Tipping, 'In Black and White', *Herald*, 5 October 1954.
52 Interview with Val Smorgon, 29 March 2006.
53 Ibid.
54 John Larkin, 'The Gentle Art of Making Millions', *The Age*, 13 September 1975.
55 'The Village of the Damned', *The Age*, 12 April 1975.
56 Interview with Ralph Dawson, 6 August 2007.
57 Helen Thomas, 'A New Era at Kew', *The Age*, 5 October 1977.

Chapter 9: Kew Salute

1 Interview with Eric Cunningham Dax, 9 January 2006.
2 Interview with Michael Glenister, 15 November 2005.
3 Interview with Julie Carpenter, 24 January 2006.
4 Interview with Max Jackson, 25 January 2006.
5 Interview with John Wakefield, 15 March 2006.
6 Interview with Julie Carpenter.
7 Interview with Patrick Reed, 3 August 2007.
8 For information on institutional violence see the first report of the Senate Inquiry into Children in Institutional Care, *Forgotten Australians: A Report on Australians who Experienced Institutional or Out-of-home Care as Children*, Chapter 4, August 2004, <http://www.aph.gov.au/SEnate/committee/clac_ctte/inst_care/report/c04.htm> (last accessed 10 January 2008).
9 Interview with Fran van Brummelen, 30 August 2005.
10 Interview with Michael Glenister.
11 Focus Group with Community Visitors, 20 June 2006.
12 Interview with Max Jackson.
13 Interview with Kurt and Maria Kraushofer, 28 March 2006.
14 Interview with John Wakefield.
15 Interview with John (Jack) and Margaret Cotter, 6 March 2006.
16 Meeting and interview with Patrick Reed, 3 August 2007.
17 Ibid.
18 Ibid.
19 Ibid.
20 Interview with Edward (Ted) Rowe, 20 April 2006.
21 Ibid.
22 Henry Reynolds, 'Violence in Australian History' in Duncan Chappell, Peter Grabowsky et al (eds), *Australian Violence: Contemporary Perspectives*, Canberra, Australian Institute of Criminology, 1991, p 17. For a discussion of masculinity and violence see Victor Seidler, 'Masculinity and Violence' in Larry May, Robert Strikwerda et al (eds), *Rethinking Masculinity: Philosophical Explorations in Light of Feminism*, Lanham, Rowman & Littlefield Inc, 1996, pp 63–75.
23 Interview with John Wakefield.
24 Interview with Fran van Brummelen.

25 Interview with Clare Turner, 5 August 2005.
26 Interview with Michael Glenister.
27 Interview with Julie Carpenter.
28 Interview with Max Jackson.
29 Ibid.
30 Interview with Jan Sharp, 10 January 2006.
31 Interview with Helen Wilson, 8 March 2006.
32 Ibid.
33 Interview with John Wakefield.
34 Interview with Clare Turner.
35 Ibid.
36 Interview with Ralph Dawson, also present Andrew Ledwidge, 3 August 2006.
37 Interview with Kurt and Maria Kraushofer.
38 Interview with Fran van Brummelen.
39 Interview with Michael Glenister.
40 Interview with Emily and Melanie Shield, 10 November 2006.
41 Interview with Kurt and Maria Kraushofer.
42 Ibid.
43 Interview with Rosalie Trower, 21 June 2006.
44 Ibid.
45 Interview between Cliff Judge and Ted Wilson, circa 1987, Kew Cottages Historical Society.
46 Interview with Jack and Margaret Cotter.
47 Ibid.
48 Interview with Emily and Melanie Shield.
49 Ibid.
50 Focus Group with Community Visitors.
51 Interview with Alma Adams, 14 August 2006.
52 Interview with Emily and Melanie Shield.
53 Interview with John Wakefield.

Chapter 10: 'Walking Ghosts'

1 For information on the impact on Victorian safety standards and deinstitutionalisation see Ian Freckelton, 'Institutional Death: The Coronial Inquest into the Deaths of Nine Men with Intellectual Disabilities', in Kelley Johnson and Rannveig Traustadóttir (eds), *Deinstitutionalization and People with Intellectual Disabilities: In and Out of Institutions*, London, Jessica Kingsley Publishers, 2005, pp 76–84; Charles Fox, 'Debating Deinstitutionalisation: The Fire at Kew Cottages in 1996 and the Idea of Community', *Health and History*, vol 5, no 2 (2003), pp 37–59.

2 Graeme Johnstone, *Inquest Findings, Comments and Recommendations into Fire and Nine Deaths at Kew Residential Services on 8 April 1996*, Melbourne, Victorian Coroner's Office, 1997.

3 Ibid, pp 33–128.

4 Ronald Haines, written submission, Kew Cottages History Project, La Trobe University, 2006.

5 Ibid.

6 Witness statement of Michael Giacomi, 'Investigation into Fatal Fire at Kew Residential Services on 8th April, 1996', prepared by Victoria Police Arson Squad, Folio 2.

7 Johnstone, p 229.

8 Haines.

9 Interview with Peter O'Connor, 2 June 2006.

10 Ibid.

11 Tony Armour quoted in 'Nine Die in Dorm Fire', *Herald Sun*, 9 April 1996, p 1.

12 Interview with Peter O'Connor.

13 Ibid.

14 Ibid.

15 Copy of letter to Jeff Kennett and signed petition, 24 April 1996, papers in the possession of Kew Cottages Parents' Association.

16 Interview with John Kelleher, 19 July 2006.

17 Ibid.

18 Ibid.

19 Interview with Jan Sharp, 17 January 2006.

20 Freckelton, p 78.

21 Johnstone, pp 232–63.

22 Interview with John Kelleher.

23 Interview with Julie Carpenter, 24 January 2006.

24 Witness statements of Chea Earpeng and Muharem Sen, 'Investigation into Fatal Fire at Kew Residential Services on 8th April, 1996', prepared by Victoria Police Arson Squad, Folio 2.

25 Interview with Helen Wilson, 8 March 2006.

26 Ibid.

27 Ibid.

28 Interview with Julie Carpenter.

29 Interview with Ralph Dawson, 6 August 2007.

30 Interview with Julie Carpenter.

31 Interview with Michael Glenister, 15 November 2005.

32 Interview with Hilda Logan, 20 March 2006.

33 Interview with Rosalie Trower, 21 June 2006.

34 Ibid.

35 Interview with Geoffrey and Elsie Welchman, 11 January 2006.

36 'Claims Quality of Life Worse than Jail', *Herald Sun*, 10 April 1996, p 3.

37 'Disaster was "Avoidable"', *The Age*, 10 April 1996, p 1; Mark Coulton, 'Kennett Faces Pressure over Blaze', *Sydney Morning Herald*, 10 April 1996, p 5.

38 Johnstone, pp 12, 315–40.

39 Ibid, p 12.

40 'With Every Ending There is a New Beginning', the memorial service for the victims of the Kew Cottages fire, Sacred Heart Church, Cotham Road, Kew, 8 April 1997, papers in the possession of the Kew Cottages Parents' Association.

Chapter 11: Bye-Bye Charlie

1 *The Kew Residential Services Redevelopment: Developing a Detailed Site Plan*, Melbourne, Victorian Government Department of Human Services, 2003, p 3.

2 Kenneth Davidson, 'Bracks Should Think Again on Kew Cottages', *The Age*, Opinion section, 12 June 2003.

3 Barbara Carter, 'We Must do Better by Those in our Care', *The Age*, Opinion section, 19 August 2003.

4 Interview with Alma Adams, 14 August 2006.

5 Sherryl Garbutt, 'Residents Deserve Better than Outdated Kew Cottages', *The Age*, Opinion section, 17 June 2003.

6 Office of the Public Advocate, *Annual Review, 2002/03*, p 5.

7 Interview with Mary Scully, 23 August 2005.

8 Interview with Rosalie Trower, 21 June 2006.

9 Ibid.

10 Carter.

11 Interview with Hilda Logan, 20 March 2006.

12 Interview with Geoffrey and Elsie Welchman, 11 January 2006.

13 Interview with Hilda Logan.

14 Ibid.

15 Interview with Geoffrey and Elsie Welchman.

16 Interview with Alma Adams.

17 Interview with Max Jackson, 25 January 2006.

18 Interview with Raymond Bouker, 14 August 2006.

19 Interview with Wendy Pennycuick, 19 December 2006.

20 Interview with Donald Starick, 21 June 2006.

21 Interview with Patty Rodgers, 29 June 2006.

22 Interview with David Honner, 4 August 2007.

23 Interview with Barry Evans, 26 July 2006.

24 Focus Group with Community Visitors, 20 June 2006.

25 Interview with Michael Glenister, 13 December 2005.

26 Ibid.

27 Interview with Patty Rodgers.

28 Interview with Raymond Bouker, 6 September 2006.

29 Interview with David Honner.

30 Ibid.

31 Interview with Ralph Dawson, 3 August 2006.

32 Interview with Raymond Bouker, 6 September 2006.

33 David Hopkins, 'Intervention Design', unpublished presentation, Action Zones – Every School is a Great School Conference, 13 September 2007, Melbourne, Australia.

Bibliography

The notes in each chapter detail the archival, official, press and manuscript material on which this book is based. The following is a list of interviews and selected secondary materials that informed the production of this history.

Kew Cottages Oral History Project Interviews

Alma Adams, 14 August 2006.
Ruth Anghie, 27 March 2006.
Sylvia Babic, 18 January 2006.
Raymond Bouker, 14 August 2006 and 6 September 2006.
Philip Brady, 9 November 2006 and 25 January 2007.
Julie Carpenter, 24 January 2006.
Charles Clark, 2 March 2006.
Robyn Cook, 1 March 2006.
John and Margaret Cotter, 6 March 2006.
James and Anna Davison, 15 March 2006.
Ralph Dawson, 3 August 2006 and 6 August 2007.
Eric Cunningham Dax, 9 January 2006 and 23 January 2006.
George and Olive Earl, 5 June 2006.
Barry Evans, 26 July 2006.
Focus Group with Community Visitors, 20 June 2006.

John Foster, 10 October 2006.
Michael Glenister, 15 November 2005 and 13 December 2005.
John Goddard, 29 May 2006.
David Honner, 12 April 2007 and 4 August 2007.
Max Jackson, 25 January 2006.
John Kelleher, 19 July 2006.
Nick Konstantaras, 15 June 2006.
Kurt and Maria Kraushofer, 28 March 2006.
Andrew Ledwidge, 31 August 2006, 26 October 2006 and 6 December 2006.
Hilda Logan, 20 March 2006.
Malcolm Macmillan, 9 March 2006.
Rose Miller, 7 March 2006.
Saral Nathaniel, 27 October 2005.
Peter O'Connor, 2 June 2006.
Wendy Pennycuick, 19 December 2006 and 4 August 2007.
Lois Philmore, 25 January 2007.
David Pitt, 19 September 2005.
Patrick Reed, 21 March 2006, 5 April 2006, 17 May 2007 and 3 August 2007.
Patricia Rodgers, 29 June 2006.
Edward Rowe, 20 April 2006.
James Scannell, 13 December 2006.
Mary Scully, 23 August 2005.
Jan Sharp, 10 January 2006 and 17 January 2006.

Emily and Melanie Shield, 10 November
2006.
Val Smorgon, 23 April 2006.
Donald Starick, 21 June 2006 and
6 December 2006.
David Sykes, 16 October 2006.
Rosalie Trower, 21 June 2006.
Clare Turner, 5 August 2005 and 10 April
2006.
Fran van Brummelen, 30 August 2005.
John Wakefield, 15 March 2006.
Christine Walton, 27 February 2006.
Steven Wears, 24 June 2006 and 7 June
2007.
Geoffrey and Elsie Welchman,
11 January 2006.
William Westgarth, 19 January 2006.
Helen Wilson, 8 March 2006.

Kew Cottages Historical Society Oral History Project

Cliff Judge and Margaret McDonald,
circa 1987.
Cliff Judge and Ted Wilson, circa 1987.
Julie McInnes and Evelyn Richards,
September 1987.
Fran van Brummelen and Irene Harvey,
17 August 1987.
Fran van Brummelen and Austra
Kurzeme, 3 and 10 September 1987.

Selected Books and Articles

Atkinson, Dorothy, Jackson, Mark and
Walmsley, Jan, *Forgotten Lives.
Exploring the History of Learning
Disability*, Kidderminster, BILD
Publications, 1997.
——, McCarthy, Michelle, Walmsley,
Jan, Cooper, Mabel, Rolph, Sheena,
Aspis, Simone, Barette, Pam,
Coventry, Mary and Ferris, Gloria,
*Good Times, Bad Times: Women
with Learning Difficulties Telling
their Stories*, Kidderminster, BILD
Publications, 2000.
Axline, Virginia, *Play Therapy: The Inner
Dynamics of Childhood*, Cambridge,
Mass, Houghton Mifflin, 1947.

Barnes, Colin and Mercer, Geoff,
Disability, Cambridge, UK, Polity
Press, 2003.
——, Oliver, Michael and Barton, Len
(eds), *Disability Studies Today*,
Cambridge, UK, Polity Press, 2002.
Barton, Len (ed), *Disability and
Dependency*, London, Falmer Press,
1989.
Brigham, Lindsay, Atkinson, Dorothy,
Jackson, Mark, Rolph, Sheena
and Walmsley, Jan (eds), *Crossing
Boundaries. Change and Continuity
in the History of Learning Disability*,
Kidderminster, BILD Publications,
2000.
Brown, Hilary and Smith, Helen (eds),
*Normalisation: A Reader for the
Nineties*, London, Routledge, 1992.
Chappell, Duncan, Grabowsky,
Peter and Strang, Heather (eds),
*Australian Violence: Contemporary
Perspectives*, Canberra, Australian
Institute of Criminology, 1991.
Cocks, Errol, Fox, Charles, Brogan,
Mark and Lee, Michael (eds), *Under
Blue Skies: The Social Construction
of Intellectual Disability in
Western Australia*, Perth, Centre
for Disability Research and
Development, Faculty of Health
and Human Sciences, Edith Cowan
University, 1996.
Coleborne, Catharine and MacKinnon,
Dolly (eds), *Madness in Australia:
Histories, Heritage and the Asylum*,
St Lucia, Qld, University of
Queensland Press in association
with the API Network and Curtin
University of Technology, 2003.
Dax, Eric Cunningham, *Asylum to
Community: The Development of the
Mental Hygiene Service in Victoria,
Australia*, Melbourne, FW Cheshire,
1961.
Ellery, Reginald, *The Cow Jumped
Over the Moon: Private Papers
of a Psychiatrist*, Melbourne,
FW Cheshire, 1956.
Fox, Charles, 'Debating
Deinstitutionalisation: The Fire at
Kew Cottages in 1996 and the Idea
of Community', *Health and History*,
vol 5, no 2 (2003), pp 37–59.
Fulcher, Gillian, *Disabling Policies? A
Comparative Approach to Education
Policy and Disability*, London,
Falmer Press, 1989.

Godwin, Louise and Wade, Catherine, *Kew Cottages Parents' Association: The First Fifty Years*, Melbourne, Kew Cottages Parents' Association Inc, 2007.

Goffman, Erving, *Asylums: Essays on the Social Situation of Mental Patients and Other Inmates*, New York, Anchor Books, 1961.

Goggin, Gerard and Newell, Christopher, *Disability in Australia: Exposing a Social Apartheid*, Sydney, UNSW Press, 2005.

Gray, Barry and Ridden, Geoff, *Lifemaps of People with Learning Disabilities*, London, Jessica Kingsley Publishers, 1988.

Hammerton, A James and Thomson, Alistair, *Ten Pound Poms: Australia's Invisible Migrants*, Manchester, Manchester University Press, 2005.

Johnson, Kelley and Traustadóttir, Rannveig (eds), *Deinstitutionalization and People with Intellectual Disabilities: In and Out of Institutions*, London, Jessica Kingsley Publishers, 2005.

Jones, Maxwell, *Therapeutic Community*, New York, Basic Books, 1953.

Judge, Astrid, 'Reflections, Memories and Sources: Growing Up at Kew Cottages', *Health and History*, vol 9, issue 1 (2007) <http://www.historycooperative.org/journals/hah/9.1/judge.html> (last accessed 10 January 2008).

Judge, Cliff and van Brummelen, Fran, *Kew Cottages: The World of Dolly Stainer*, Melbourne, Spectrum Publications, 2002.

Kugel, Robert and Wolfensberger,

Wolf (eds), *Changing Patterns in Residential Services for the Mentally Retarded*, Washington, President's Committee on Mental Retardation, 1969.

Lloyd, Arthur, *Payment By Results: Kew Cottages First 100 Years 1887–1987*, Melbourne, Kew Cottages and St Nicholas Parents' Association Inc, 1987.

May, Larry, Strikwerda, Robert and Hopkins, Patrick (eds), *Rethinking Masculinity: Philosophical Explorations in Light of Feminism*, Lanham, Rowman & Littlefield Inc, 1996.

Paris, Chris, *Housing Australia*, Melbourne, Macmillan Education Australia Pty Ltd, 1993.

Pitt, David Buxton, *For the Love of the Children: My Life and Medical Career*, Melbourne, Pitt Publishing, 1999.

Rapley, Mark, *The Social Construction of Intellectual Disability*, Cambridge, UK, Cambridge University Press, 2004.

Rolph, Sheena, Atkinson, Dorothy, Nind, Melanie and Welshman, John, *Witnesses to Change: Families, Learning Difficulties and History*, Kidderminster, BILD Publications, 2005.

Shakespeare, Tom, Gillespie-Sells, Kath and Davies, Dominic, *The Sexual Politics of Disability: Untold Desires*, London, Cassell, 1996.

Wolfensberger, Wolf, *Normalization: The Principle of Normalization in Human Services*, Toronto, National Institute on Mental Retardation, 1972.

Index